Praise for CLIFF AND through Cancer and Beyond

"A real-life journey into love, separation, and the reality of cancer impacting our companion animals. JoAnne DeFluri and Cliff take us inside their lives to teach us about the struggles, smiles, and mutual support these best friends gave each other. A beautiful story of unconditional love and loyalty."

—**Mary Hessler Key,** PhD,
author of *What Animals Teach Us*

"As a pet owner myself who has seen several beloved cats through cancer, I identified with your story personally. I can see social workers at veterinary hospitals and veterinarians throughout the country using this book as a resource for their clients who are themselves mourning the illness or death of a beloved pet. It is both informative and touching."

—**Nancy L. Eaton,** Dean of University Libraries,
The Pennsylvania State University

"An honest and emotional account of one woman's journey through love and loss, *Cliff and I* will resonate with readers who have struggled to navigate the medical maze of caring for their pets through the ravages of cancer and beyond."

—**Gary Kowalski,** author of *The Souls of Animals* and
Goodbye Friend: Healing Wisdom For Anyone Who Has Ever Lost A Pet

CLIFF AND I

MY DOG'S JOURNEY
THROUGH CANCER AND BEYOND

CLIFF AND I

MY DOG'S JOURNEY
THROUGH CANCER AND BEYOND

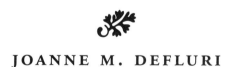

JOANNE M. DEFLURI

PUBLISHING WORKS
Exeter, New Hampshire

Front cover photo by Lettie Davis.
Book design by Lauren Hawkins.

The author may be contacted at CliffandI2006@aol.com and please visit her website at www.CliffandI.com.

PublishingWorks
60 Winter Street
Exeter, NH 03833
800/333-9883
www.publishingworks.com

Marketing and Sales:
Revolution Booksellers
800/738-6603
www.revolutionbooksellers.com

Library of Congress Cataloging-in-Publication Data
DeFluri, JoAnne M., 1960–
     Cliff and I: My dog's journey through cancer and beyond /
JoAnne M. DeFluri.
          p. cm.
          ISBN 1–933002–19–0 (pbk.)
1. Dogs--Diseases. 2. Cancer in animals. 3. Veterinary oncology.
4. DeFluri, JoAnne M., 1960– 5. Human-animal relationships.
I. Title: Cliff and I. II. Title.
          SF992.C35D44 2006
          636.7'0896994--dc22
                                                  2005055987

Printed in Canada

For Jokonita and Drake,
who continue to inspire me

but most of all,
for Cliff, who spoke no words
but through his eyes, he taught me life.
Silence crossed boundaries and love grew.
Godspeed, my friend.

Contents

Acknowledgments xi

Foreword xv

Preface xvii

1 Our Life: October 2000 1

2 Cliff aus der Eremitenklause: January 1997 7

3 Jokonita vom Christinen Brunnen: October 1999 15

4 Finding the Lump: July and August 2000 19

5 The Diagnosis: August and September 2000 25

6 Saving Cliff: September 2000 29

7 Banking Cliff's Sperm: September 2000 39

8 Radiation Therapy: October 2000 43

9 A Twist of Fate: November 2000 57

10 Chemotherapy and Pamidronate: December 2000 75

11 Acupuncture and Reiki: December 2000 81

12 Our Return to Pennsylvania—Cliff Romps Again: April 2001 91

13 Spondylosis: July 2001 97

14 One-Year Anniversary: Summer and Fall 2001 103

15 A Turn of Events: December 2001 111

16 Bringing Cliff Home: January 2002 125

17 The Next Steps: Winter 2002 131

18 Life as We Know It: Spring and Summer 2002 137

Afterword 141

Resources 149

About the Author 153

Acknowledgments

There are many people who have helped me complete this journey, and first and foremost is my dear husband, Dick. During all the months that I spent in Colorado while Cliff was being treated for cancer, Dick never once complained. He never questioned my choices, and always supported me.

Dr. Bonita Selting provided guidance and editing expertise as I prepared the manuscript for publication. Thank you for helping to make this project a reality.

Jeremy Townsend, my publisher, believed in our story from day one. Because of her, Cliff's story will live on forever. This led me to Melissa Hayes, my editor—who could have known that we would connect so quickly? She understood Cliff's story, and how important it was for me to tell it as it happened. Her expertise helped enrich our story, and I am very thankful that she has been a part of this project. Lauren Hawkins played an instrumental role as the book's designer. I thank her for designing a book that so beautifully portrays Cliff's life.

I have many friends and family members who helped me through this experience; they supported me, cried with me, and were always there. Thank you. I am especially grateful to my sister Amy and my nephew Chase, who spent many days and weeks in Fort Collins with me. Just having you there gave me something to smile about.

There are no words to express my deepest gratitude to every doctor, nurse, student, and technician who cared for Cliff. You all walk this earth with one goal in mind: to bring peace and comfort to our animal companions, and to those of us who love them.

To Cliff's primary oncologist, Dr. Kimberly Selting—thank you for always being there for us. For sixteen months you were by our sides, providing medical expertise, support, and kindness. You are more than a doctor, you are my friend. We made a great team and I am proud that you were part of our journey. Whenever I reflect on everything Cliff endured, I think of you with immense gratitude.

To Dr. Gregory Ogilvie—you were there for us, twenty-four/seven, looking for treatments that would help Cliff during those critical days. You are a wonderful doctor, a kind man, and someone I will never forget.

To Dr. Stephen Withrow—from day one, I trusted you completely. Thank you for your surgical skills and for providing wonderful doctors to care for Cliff. In doing so, you help to make the world a better place.

To Dr. Elizabeth Pluhar—you literally changed our lives by teaching us more about Cliff's disease. In the end, what you discovered gave us a new lease on life, and I will be forever grateful.

To Dr. Brenda McClelland—you have an exceptional gift, one that opened my mind to possibilities I would never have known existed. Thank you for sharing it with us.

To Dr. Narda Robinson—our talks during Cliff's acupuncture treatments gave me renewed strength to carry on. You are more than just a talented doctor; you have a kind heart and I thank you for openly sharing your thoughts with me.

To Dr. Stephen Warren, who diagnosed Cliff's cancer—you are a great doctor, and someone I can always count on. Thank you.

To Dr. Alan Friedlander—I can't thank you enough for providing excellent care for Cliff while we were in Pennsylvania, and for so capably following the CSU protocol.

To Dr. Karen Jones—thank you for caring for Cliff when we needed you.

To Dr. Debra Smart—if I had never met you, I may have never gone to CSU for Cliff's treatment. Thank you for your straightforward advice that sent us there. In doing so, my life has been changed forever.

To Dr. Sheri Beattie—you hold the future of Cliff's lineage, and one day, I hope to share the joy of his puppies with you. Thank you for being there when we needed your expertise.

To Teri Nelson—Kim and Greg urged me to talk with you for months; little did I know how much I would benefit from doing so. When I was having a difficult time, you helped me move on. Because I did, you are reading our story now.

All of you have played very special roles at different times in Cliff's care. In each of you, we found hope. Thank you!

Foreword

When I first met Cliff and JoAnne, I was immediately struck by their bond. Cliff was a majestic dog and always seemed at total peace with JoAnne. As I got to know them both separately and together, I realized that they had connected in a unique way. Cliff seemed to fill a special spot in JoAnne's heart and he was infinitely devoted to her. We embarked on a journey to fight his cancer, and were met by many unexpected obstacles along the way. It seemed like every time we felt we were near the end of treatment, we had a new problem to solve. JoAnne met each challenge head-on, strong and practical. I was always amazed at how she could keep herself together, take in all the facts, ask all the pertinent questions, and make a plan, then let herself feel all the emotions after she knew she had a path to follow. Stopping treatment was never an option so long as Cliff was still in the fight with us.

As I read this story I was reminded of all Cliff's ups and downs. JoAnne shows us the emotions and curiosity (What can be done?) of an owner caring for a beloved companion. I think each pet owner is faced with the responsibility of being the voice for his or her companion in difficult times. I am privileged to be a part of this bond at these critical moments—and it is at these very moments that I realize how much our animal companions really can "talk" to us. JoAnne has done an excellent job of letting us in on her communication with Cliff, and how she was able to be his voice in a time of need.

—**Kimberly A. Selting,** *DVM, MS*
Diplomate ACVIM (Oncology)

Preface

I never envisioned that one day, I would write a book . . . but that was before I had a story to tell. Living through the experience of my dog Cliff's battle with cancer, I found my inner voice—a part of myself that I never knew existed. Since Cliff was not able to speak for himself, I decided that I would do it for him.

Initially, I would sit and write during Cliff's treatments, and while I found this to be therapeutic, I had no intention of sharing his story with the world. As time went on, however, friends who read my frequent e-mails often commented on my ability to convey what we were living through. Although I shelved the story for a while, eventually I knew I had to finish it. I realized that although our experience is touched with some sadness, it's also filled with inspiration. I came to believe that sharing our story could benefit others who face the same situation.

My motivation for writing this book was twofold: first, to increase awareness of the high rate of cancer in our animal companions, and to raise money for cancer research; and second, to offer information and support to others who are on this same journey with their pets.

During the past few years, I have been contacted by many people who were looking for guidance, suggestions, and often, just someone to talk to about their experience. I was fortunate in that I had the resources to provide the care Cliff needed during his battle with cancer. I understand that each reader will have to decide, after learning what is involved, what course of action to pursue. Individual factors such as the animal's age and general health and each owner's personal feelings and beliefs will play a role in the decision-making process. It's important to decide what is best for each pet in each individual situation, and I've included a list of resources to help readers during this process.

I hope that readers will find something within these pages to provide some hope along the way; if they do, then I'll know Cliff's battle was not in vain.

—JoAnne M. DeFluri

I
Our Life

I glanced over at the clock—6:38 A.M. I rolled over and lay there for a few minutes as I let out a deep sigh and thought about the day ahead. Cliff and Jokonita were still sleeping in their beds on the floor next to me, but I knew they would want to go out soon. I slowly got out of bed and made my way to the bathroom without turning on the light, to allow them a few more minutes of sleep. I quickly washed my face and brushed my teeth. I looked in the mirror and decided to throw on a bit of powder; that would have to do it for now. As I reached to pick up their leashes, the dogs started heading for the door, knowing it was time to go.

Today was the third day I would be dropping Cliff off at the Colorado State University Veterinary Teaching Hospital for radiation therapy. We walked out the door of our hotel room, both dogs attached to their leashes—not so much to control them, but to ease the fears of anyone we happened to pass in the hallway. These two big, beautiful German shepherds were actually quite gentle, but could appear intimidating when passersby first saw them.

Cliff was the larger of the two, standing almost a head taller than Jokonita (pronounced *Ya-ka-nita*). Before Cliff was diagnosed with cancer, he weighed 106 pounds, compared to Jokonita's 74 pounds. Fortunately, Cliff had maintained his weight so far, but I knew that he could still lose a few pounds as the treatments continued. Both dogs were very athletic, with little to no excess body fat. They had very similar coloring, mostly golden brown with reddish highlights and accents of black on their backs, often called the "saddle." Their fur was soft, and I loved snuggling with them and smelling their natural scent. Cliff had one very distinguishing characteristic—a black star in the middle of his forehead. Their big

I

brown eyes melted my heart when I looked into them, seeing there the reflection of the love we shared.

We walked around outside for a while as they sniffed the grass, finding the perfect spot to leave their mark. I noticed that the clouds were hanging low in the sky, and that there was a light mist in the air as fog hid the mountains. I realized then that I was still very tired. I hadn't been sleeping well lately. I knew this would not go on forever; I just needed to hang in there for Cliff.

As I opened up the back doors of the Suburban, Cliff and Jokonita jumped in together. I walked around to the driver's side and let myself in. When I glanced at the clock, I saw that it was 7:15 A.M. *We should have plenty of time to get to the VTH by 7:30,* I thought. With the light morning traffic, my drive up College Avenue to West Drake Road took just a few minutes. As I pulled into the parking lot, I felt nauseous and tense, just as I'd been feeling the past two mornings. I got out and walked around to the back of the car. I could sense that Jokonita didn't want Cliff to go in alone.

"I'll be right back, Nita girl," I said softly. "Please stay here and wait for me."

I attached Cliff's leash to his brass choker collar, and we walked across the parking lot, stopping at the small patch of grass outside the front door. Cliff had made it a ritual to mark this spot each morning.

Today was his third day of treatments, and although I'd been hoping we would start to develop a routine, this was still very new to us. We walked in, and I looked around the waiting area; it was nearly empty. I took a seat, the same one I'd occupied for the last two days, and Cliff sat down next to me. I leaned down to hug him, telling him that it was going to be okay, and that I loved him very much.

We were soon greeted by Amy, a senior veterinary student, and we talked briefly as I took off Cliff's collar and leash. Amy handed me a soft, red fabric leash, and I slipped it over Cliff's head. I hugged him again, and kissed the black star on the top of his forehead. I stroked his ears, soft as velvet, and whispered, "It's going to be okay . . . I'll be here waiting for you when you're done." I handed the leash to Amy, knowing that I was now facing the hardest part of the day. Cliff looked up at me with his big brown eyes, as if to say, *Please don't leave.* My heart ached. I encouraged him to go with Amy as I fought back the tears. I walked around the corner to get quickly out of sight. I didn't want Cliff to see the pain I was feeling. I needed to be strong for him.

As I walked out the door, tears streaming down my face, I knew that I had to calm down before I got back to Jokonita. I took a few deep breaths and tried to steady myself, standing there staring into space, oblivious to anything around me. I slowly regained my composure, walked back to the Suburban, and saw that Nita was now between the two middle seats, watching for my return. As I opened the door, she reached up and planted a wet kiss on my cheek. I stroked her head and told her that all was well—we'd be back for Cliff in a little while. I knew that it would actually be hours before we returned, and I silently hoped that those hours would fly by quickly.

I pulled out of the parking lot and decided to go to a nearby park so Jokonita could get some exercise. I'd only been in Fort Collins for a few days, but I'd learned my way around well enough to find some quiet places where the dogs could run and play freely. As I pulled into the park, Jokonita was looking out the window, excited to see where we were. She jumped out with a red rubber Frisbee already in her mouth. Designed with dogs in mind, these special Frisbees have a raised "dog bone" in the middle that makes it easy for dogs to pick them up with their teeth. I grabbed another one and threw it for her to chase. The dogs and I often played this game for hours, Cliff and Jokonita running side by side with Frisbees in their mouths, trying to be first to the one that I'd thrown. I would throw it on an angle so that it landed on its side and rolled on the grass like a wheel, the dogs chasing it until it fell flat onto the grass.

3

When they reached it, they'd keep the one they carried tightly clasped in their mouth, pointing it toward the one that I just threw. Sometimes while playing they would pick up the Frisbee by the raised bone on the top, or sometimes bend it in half, carrying it as easily as I would carry a piece of bread.

It was good to have Jokonita with me. The diversion helped to take my mind off why we were really there. After about an hour, we worked our way back to the car. I reached inside to get a water bowl and some water for Jokonita, which she quickly lapped up. It had been a quiet morning, with only a few other people walking their dogs in the distance. I decided that we should go back to the hotel, and as soon as I opened the door, Nita jumped in.

The Marriott Residence Inn would become our home for the next four weeks while we were in town for Cliff's radiation treatments. It could be even longer if the doctors determined that Cliff would need chemotherapy following the radiation.

We got back to the hotel, and as soon as I opened the door to our room, I collapsed onto the bed. I felt completely exhausted, emotionally drained. I'd planned to go out on my road bike at some point, but the weather was still slightly overcast, and I didn't really feel like going right then. I picked up my cell phone and dialed a few numbers, looking for someone to talk to—someone who would possibly understand what we were going through. I had no luck, just getting voice mail, so I set the phone down. I'd have to try again later.

I decided I might as well go out and brave the light drizzle. I knew I wouldn't feel any better just lying around moping. I quickly changed into my biking clothes, got my bike ready, and pushed it to the door. Jokonita walked over to inspect.

"I'm just going out for a quick ride," I said. "I'll be back soon."

I wasn't exactly sure where this ride would take me, but thought I'd head toward Boyd Lake. I had found the lake the first time I'd come to Fort Collins, and this was the spot where I took Cliff and Jokonita each day after Cliff's treatment. I felt a sense of calmness there, and I thought Cliff and Jokonita could feel it too. It was a beautiful, peaceful lake, not as busy this time of year with boats or Jet Skis. Usually there were only a few lonely fishermen out on the water. It was the perfect place for us to spend the afternoons together, and I fed them their dinner there. Sometimes we stayed long into the evening to watch the sun set over the mountain.

Although I felt tired, I really needed to ride. I had a lot of anger and fear inside of me, and I hoped to leave some of it on the road. As I pedaled along, I started to feel some of the load lifting. The faster I went, the better I felt. I knew that I was now on a mission to escape. I hardly paid any attention to the traffic, focusing on the open road in front of me. As I headed out of the residential area and into farmland, I started to take in the lovely surroundings. I'd always been a very optimistic person, and I realized that there was beauty to be found, even in this gray, gloomy day.

I took the turn off the highway that led to the bike path, and followed along until I reached the lake. I noticed that the leaves had started to change color since the last time I'd been there, and with each breath I inhaled, I felt the freshness of the rain. As I continued my ride, I felt a strength that I had been sorely lacking in recent days surging through me.

Suddenly, I was overwhelmed with the feeling that I should tell our story. I knew beyond a doubt that what Cliff and I were experiencing, as painful as it might be, would mold me for the rest of my life. The harder I pedaled, the more inspired I became. Although I had never considered myself to be the literary type, I felt strongly that our story might benefit someone else. There would be lessons learned along the way, I was sure of that; maybe by sharing what we were going through, I would be able to help others.

As I rode along the bike path, my speed ever quickening, I was flooded with memories—reflections of what we'd gone through in the past several months. I felt heartened by my resolution.

Cliff and I had a story to tell.

2
Cliff aus der Eremitenklause

Cliff aus der Eremitenklause, as his pedigree reads, came into our lives in January 1997. We had decided six months earlier that we wanted to add a dog to our family to keep me company while my husband, Dick, was traveling. Dick's work in the financial industry involved frequent trips throughout Pennsylvania and the East Coast to see clients, attend conferences, or meet with his business partners. While I never really minded his time away from home, we felt that a dog would make a good companion for me.

During the past four years, my sister Amy had been living with us while she attended Penn State. Amy and I were more than just sisters. Although there was an eleven-year age difference between us, we were very close and enjoyed doing things together. Our mother had died suddenly when Amy was only five years old, and for a number of years I helped to care for her and my younger brothers. I was still in high school at the time, and we endured some challenging years together, all of which brought us even closer. Knowing that Amy was getting ready to graduate from college soon, I agreed with Dick that the timing was right. I was very excited, but also a bit apprehensive.

Dick and I had talked to Bob Martin, a two-time National Champion at the German Shepherd Nationals, who would become our personal dog trainer. Years before I had met Dick, he had raised two Rottweilers, and had enlisted Bob's help with their training. Dick and I felt comfortable that Bob would find the right dog for us.

One day Bob called and told us he had found the perfect dog: an adult male German shepherd from Germany named Cliff, who was five years old at the time. Bob had traveled to Germany and personally handpicked Cliff. He knew the kennel where Cliff had been raised. Apparently the

7

owners were in some sort of financial bind and had decided to sell him. Later, as I grew to know and love Cliff, it was hard to imagine the heartache it must have caused to those who had to sell him.

Cliff's lineage went way back, and his ancestors were World Champion Siegers. In Germany, that title was reserved for the male or female adult German shepherd (over two years of age) who was named that year's Grand Champion—in German, *Sieger* (male) or *Siegerin* (female). Cliff had received extensive training and was a Shutzhund III, a term I knew nothing about at the time. I soon learned that to earn the title of Shutzhund III, a dog must be proficient in three categories; obedience, tracking, and protection. Many Shutzhund III dogs become police dogs, while others provide personal protection or serve as companions—ideal positions for dogs of such formidable presence. At the time, I didn't think I needed a dog with such intelligence and skills; I simply wanted a companion, someone who would become a part of our family. I had no idea before I met Cliff that dogs are really a lot like us. If you give them love and care, they will forever be at your side, always your most loyal friend.

When Bob brought Cliff to our house, I remember being surprised at how big he was (close to 100 pounds). But it was more than just his size. His mere presence commanded respect. He was very regal-looking as he sat next to Bob, straight and tall, almost as if he had been ordered to sit at attention. Despite his size and powerful aura, however, I never felt intimidated by him. I saw the softness in his eyes. In the days to come, I was to discover that my initial impressions were correct.

Bob told us that Cliff had been trained in German, and gave us a cheat sheet so that we would be able to learn the German commands. I will never forget those first few days. Cliff would listen to our somewhat clumsy commands in the mumbled German that we used. He would follow us outside, very calm, but at the same time remaining quite aloof. He seemed content enough to be there with us. When we were in the house, he would mainly stay in the living room, which is centrally located. In the early days, he never wanted to sleep in my bedroom; if he did follow me in when I went to bed, later in the night I would hear him get up and go back out to the living room. It was as if he thought his sole purpose was to guard the house. I assumed he had been doing this his whole life, and that perhaps he didn't yet understand he had a different role now. The first few weeks, he never barked or showed any sign of aggression. He was simply there, and stayed because he was told to do so.

In the weeks that followed, I was the one who spent the most time with Cliff. When Dick was working and traveling, it was just Cliff and me. I would load him up in the 4Runner and we would drive to different places and go hiking. He would do whatever I asked of him, and although my German was not the best, we somehow learned to communicate. He came to understand English, and as time progressed, Dick and I spoke more English than German in our daily routines. I learned that *nein* in German was "no," and Cliff learned that "no" in English meant *nein*. Mostly though, I spoke to him as if he were a human being who could understand what I was saying. I think my body language and my actions played a big role in our learning to communicate with each other. He learned to drink water out of a sports cap, trusting the very first time I held it for him that I wouldn't splash him. We would take breaks while on hikes and sit next to each other. I would feed him pieces of beef jerky, which he'd gently take from my hand with teeth I knew could just as easily have taken my arm off.

His size did intimidate more than a few, and on one particular hike a bow hunter dressed in camouflage called out to let me know he was there. I guessed that he did not want to surprise Cliff. Always a little leery of hunters, I now felt a sense of empowerment having Cliff by my side. Being a female alone in the woods was not something I would have to worry about again. Cliff seemed to like being in the mountains with me, and I enjoyed our early days together, exploring our surroundings and getting to know each other.

The weeks turned into months, and one day when we were driving back from a hike, it happened—Cliff barked. We had just passed a truck with a dog leaning out the window, and as we drove by, Cliff suddenly barked. Up until this time, he'd been such a quiet animal. While he accompanied me everywhere, he had never made a sound. I remembered that Bob had said Cliff would let us know when he had accepted us. Did this mean we were his pack now?

In the following weeks, Cliff showed signs that he had indeed accepted us as his family, especially me. He started to sleep in my bedroom, and even got up on the bed after some initial coaxing. I guessed that he had been trained to *not* get up on the furniture. He would follow me from room to room and lie next to me wherever I went. He became my shadow. Regardless of what I was doing, I would look at him and talk to him, fully knowing that he did not yet understand everything I was saying. But he was starting to respond to my loving gestures. He became more affectionate, and would put his head under my hand to let me know he wanted to be petted. I would hug him and kiss his forehead, telling him that I didn't know how I had gone so long without him in my life. I had fallen in love with this amazing creature. It was a different type of love—one in which neither of us asked anything of the other except to simply be together. I went from not having a dog to never wanting to be away from Cliff.

Our relationship was further strengthened when we took spontaneous breaks from our daily routine. At times we would stop for a dip in a stream, Cliff jumping playfully through the water while I walked along the banks, trying to stay dry. Sometimes, for no particular reason, we would pause at a mountain overlook, where we'd sit on the grass and look out at the vista below, enjoying the beautiful bird song around us. At times like these, I would sit very close to Cliff and gently massage his neck and back. He seemed to love the extra attention, and our relationship grew ever stronger.

Our daily hikes often involved an object as simple as a stick. It turned a casual walk into an enticing game of strategy, as I methodically threw the stick for Cliff and he brought it back to me, placing it gently at my feet.

We had another favorite game that I simply called "kick." Sometimes the object that became our ball was actually a round stone, a large black walnut still in its outer green shell, or an apple from the orchard that had fallen to the ground. I would kick the object and Cliff would chase it, most times not picking it up with his mouth but just following it, staring intensely at the stone or walnut until I kicked it again. He would sometimes pick up an apple, and as he bit into it with his powerful jaws, it would split into pieces. I would notice a twinkle of surprise in his eyes as he tasted the tart fruit. I would often pick up a piece of the apple and munch along with him.

These simple pleasures brought us both so much joy, and served to reinforce our growing bond.

Football season was fast approaching, and soon Cliff would get to meet my extended "family." I was sure that everyone would quickly take to him, as he seemed to have that effect on people. We entertained a lot, because Dick is a Penn State alumnus and many of his fraternity brothers return for the games. They, along with their wives, spend long weekends with us, some staying in our house and others staying in our guesthouse by the pool. This would be a test of Cliff's social skills. It was important that he get to know our friends and understand that they were allowed to be inside our fenced-in yard. Things went smoothly from the beginning, and each weekend Cliff got to meet new people. Some took to him more than others—usually the women, as Cliff had an undeniable charm about him. I think some of the men were initially intimidated by his size, but they soon came around once they realized what a gentle creature he was. Cliff was a puppy at heart, and just happened to be living in a very large body.

From the day Cliff came to live with us, Dick would work him a few times a week by doing a series of drills in the backyard. These were mostly obedience exercises designed to encourage Cliff to remain in one place for a period of time, until he was given the command to move. Cliff did his part, smoothly going through the motions, as I'm sure he'd done during the years he lived in Germany. But Cliff's role was not the same now; he was no longer being asked to track and search for items. His primary task was to be my companion, and it was one that he quickly adjusted to. I think these drills were initially intended to let Cliff know that Dick was his master, but in the end, it did not turn out like that. Cliff clearly came to see *me* as his master, although I never thought of myself that way. I thought of Cliff as my equal; he just happened to have four legs instead of two.

One evening we were hosting a dinner party in our backyard for the Paterno Library at Penn State, of which Dick is a board member. The guests were donors and potential donors to the library, most of whom I did not know well. None of them had ever met Cliff before, so I was interested to see how the evening would go. As it turned out, Cliff stole the show! He went from table to table, greeting each guest. A few days later I received numerous thank-you cards, among them one that I will never forget. A woman wrote that she'd had a wonderful time at our house, but had been most impressed with Cliff; she had never met a dog with a personality like his. I guess others were starting to notice what I had seen in Cliff all along.

As we entered the heart of football season, Cliff became good friends with the staff of La Purple Chef, especially Chef Marco and Cori, who prepared catered dinners in our home. Chef Marco and Cori would arrive hours in advance to prep the food and set up for the evening. Cliff would often hang out in the kitchen, looking for delectable morsels. Marco appreciated the fact that Cliff enjoyed his cuisine, especially his spiced-seared filet tips with creamy risotto, smothered in mushroom gravy. My stepson Blake also got into the act, baking batches of biscuits for Cliff as a special treat. Cliff would wait patiently while they baked and then eat them warm, right from the oven.

As time went on, more and more people grew to love Cliff, and appreciate his loving nature. When I look back at pictures from every party and every dinner we had at our home during this time, Cliff is in all of them, sitting right next to me—sometimes even wearing a paper chef's hat on his head.

Cliff had not only become my ideal companion—he had fully immersed himself into our lifestyle. I found it difficult to remember what life had been like before Cliff came along.

3
Jokonita vom Christinen Brunnen

A couple of years after Cliff joined our family, I was talking to Jackie, who worked with Bob, our dog-trainer friend. I mentioned that if she ever found the right female German shepherd, I would like to breed Cliff. It wasn't long before Jackie called me from Germany to say she had found the perfect match for Cliff. I realized that she had misunderstood me; I had wanted a puppy of Cliff's, not another adult dog. But that quickly changed as Jackie told me how beautiful Jokonita was, and what an ideal mate she would be for Cliff. She said they would have beautiful puppies together. It took me just a moment to absorb what she was telling me. Soon I had agreed, and asked her to go ahead and get Jokonita for us.

Jokonita had to stay in Germany for a short while longer, as she'd recently given birth to a litter. Because she was a show dog, she needed to win another show in order to give her puppies the recognition they were due. I agreed, and a few months later Jokonita arrived.

The day that Jackie delivered Jokonita to us, I was outside playing with Cliff. After letting the two dogs sniff each other through the fence, I opened the gate and in ran Jokonita. She and Cliff continued to sniff, and then started chasing each other, very playfully, around the yard. I quickly ran inside to get my camera, and upon my return a few seconds later, saw that Jokonita had fallen into the pool. At the time the pool had a blue bubble-type solar cover on it, and it occurred to me that she hadn't realized there was water under it. Fortunately, Blake was in the backyard with Jackie, and was able to quickly pull Jokonita to safety. When winter arrived in a few months the solar cover would be replaced by a much more substantial one that anchored to the concrete around the pool. In the meantime, I knew I'd have to keep a watchful eye on Jokonita, as well as any other dogs who might be visiting, until they realized the potential danger of getting caught up in the pool cover.

As it turned out, Nita's adventure in the pool proved to be a harbinger of things to come. She was a live wire! I will never forget those first few days after her arrival, and how at times I thought I had made a huge mistake in acquiring this new dog. The regular routine that Cliff and I had established over the years was now disrupted. When Cliff and I would go for hikes, Cliff—always off lead—would stay right with me. Not Jokonita. She was a crazy girl when she was off her leash. She would take off, chasing our cats, and the squirrels and rabbits we encountered on our hikes. After having her with me for just one day, I told Dick that I didn't feel ready for her, and somehow, she just didn't seem to fit in with us. Dick thought I should just give it more time. I really didn't want to send her back; I just didn't know how to handle her. I decided to take Dick's advice and wait to see if we could adjust to each other.

During the next few weeks when we went for hikes, I kept her on a leash. I was worried that she would run off and not be able to find her way back to us. When we went out on the mountain behind our house, on our own property, I was able to give her more freedom. As time went by, she started to stay with us more often. I learned that as soon as she got distracted by a squirrel, I would have to quickly change her mindset so she would not take off. I'd call out to her and have her sit next to me, rubbing her head and talking to her until I thought the squirrel was out of sight. Maybe being a show dog in Germany had not afforded her much time for "freedom walks" in the mountains. She was just very curious about her new environment. Nita was quick to learn from Cliff, following him around the house. I soon found that instead of having one shadow, I now had two.

While Cliff had always gotten along well with our cats—littermates Spooky, all black, and the orange one, Tigger—Nita didn't take to them quite as well. Cliff didn't mind their antics, and would even rub noses with them—but Nita only wanted to chase them. Spooky and Tigger usually preferred to be outside, and when they were inside, they had their own space. Initially, this was because of Dick's severe allergies to cats; but once Jokonita joined our family, I think the cats preferred to stay in their own place, safe from Nita's exuberant games. Fortunately for Spooky and Tigger, they could squeeze through the fence or quickly scamper up a tree to escape her attentions. Nevertheless, it was probably safe to assume that Nita had *not* been raised with cats.

Jackie assured me that trainers had linked Jokonita's aggression toward small animals to a hard-wired "prey drive" that is part of the breed. It's one thing if a dog is raised around cats, she said; but in the absence of that experience, it is the nature of the breed to chase small forest animals and cats. In days gone by, this is how dogs augmented their diets while performing shepherding duties. The shepherd often didn't have a bag of dog food in his satchel, and food was hard to come by, even for him; thus, the dog was often expected to fill in the gaps in his diet. While this had never occurred to me, it made sense.

Jackie also mentioned that the same part of the dog's mind that contains the "prey drive" also holds the "play drive." Play drive is the dog's version of the human urge to play cowboys and Indians, mock war, chasing games, and so forth. The fact that Jokonita also had this very strong play drive would help to offset her prey drive. It would be my job to supply her with plenty of toys and stimulation to change her mindset, and Jokonita seemed to love playing with Cliff, so I felt confident it was an endeavor we could accomplish together.

I rarely took Cliff or Nita to a dog park, since we had so much open space to roam right near our home. The few times I did, Cliff was eager to play with dogs of all shapes and sizes, whereas Nita preferred to play only with Cliff and me. She never mingled with the other dogs, choosing to play

Frisbee with us instead. While I found this a bit odd, I again attributed it to her show dog background. Maybe she hadn't had a chance to play with many other dogs before coming to live with us.

Despite these differences, and the occasional challenge, as the weeks and months went by, I realized that I *had* done the right thing after all. While she was a lively animal, Jokonita was definitely a positive addition to our family. Cliff liked having her around, and they bonded quickly. I put their dog beds on the floor next to each other, but they would often curl up in just one bed together. I was curious about their silent form of communication and wished I was privy to their thoughts. They became very much a couple, and would roll around on the floor and play. Jokonita was very affectionate toward Cliff from the very beginning, and would lick his entire head, planting wet kisses everywhere. It gave me great joy to see the love they shared. I realized then that Cliff would have a much happier, more complete life, having a companion of his own.

4
Finding the Lump

It was the end of July, and we were heading to Colorado with much excitement and anticipation. The long-awaited day had arrived: We would be moving into our second home, in the Vail Valley.

We had been coming to Colorado for many years, mostly to ski for a few weeks each winter. Recently, we had decided to build a second home here, and now that it was completed, I knew I'd be spending months at a time here with Cliff and Jokonita. Dick still had to travel quite a bit for business, and it was reassuring to know that I'd have the dogs for company when he was away.

I had also developed a circle of friends in Colorado, and I looked forward to spending more time with them, enjoying everything the mountains of Colorado had to offer. In addition to the fabulous skiing in the winter, the summer promised hiking, fishing, rafting, and golf. (Not that I was much into golf at the time—but living in a community that had beautiful golf courses was an added plus!) Summer days in Colorado are mostly filled with clear blue skies and endless sunshine, and unlike the East Coast, there is no humidity in the mountains. I was very much looking forward to spending the next few months here.

We had left State College, Pennsylvania, on July 31, and were flying to Eagle, Colorado, in the small private plane Dick used for business travel. I felt fortunate to have this luxury, as it made traveling with two large dogs very easy. If we hadn't had access to the plane, I would have opted to drive cross-country rather than subject the dogs to flying in the baggage compartment of a commercial airliner. Of course, as generous as Dick is, he insisted we take it, saying that this was part of the reason he had the plane.

Both Cliff and Jokonita were accustomed to the plane, and when we got to the hangar, they quickly climbed the stairs and found a place on the floor next to my seat. I had spread out a fluffy blue comforter for them to lie on. As we got ready to take off, I grabbed a bag of beef jerky. When we started to gain altitude, I gave them small pieces to chew and swallow, to help their ears adjust to the change in the altitude pressure. I remembered the first time Cliff had flown on the plane. He had shaken his head after takeoff, and I realized he was just trying to adjust to the pressure. Since then, I'd made sure to have plenty of jerky with me whenever we flew.

We had about a seven-hour flight ahead of us, and would most likely be stopping halfway to refuel. As we reached our cruising altitude of 21,000 feet, Cliff and Jokonita were comfortably resting on the floor next to me, and would most likely sleep until we landed.

I couldn't wait to spend the first night in our new house, and have them there with me. I believed that we'd found the perfect place for us, and I just knew the dogs would love it too. Over the course of the next few weeks, I spent the days unpacking and taking Cliff and Jokonita for long hikes. Dick stayed with us for the first two weeks, but then headed back to Pennsylvania for business, returning again at the end of August. While he was gone, I planned to explore our corner of Colorado with Cliff and Jokonita.

I wasted no time. We started heading out together each day, often taking long drives to investigate the new and exciting areas around us. I'd load the two dogs into the Suburban—they loved riding in the car—and off we'd go. Most days, I didn't know where we were headed, never quite having a plan, just going where the road took us that particular day. We'd stop often, sometimes along the Colorado River, and I'd let them out to romp and have fun in the water. They loved this, and took every opportunity to dive in and play. Regardless of where we went, they loved to go with me, and no matter where we ended up, they were just happy to be along for the ride. I soon grew to treasure my time alone with them in this beautiful place. I knew that when they were with me, I would never feel alone.

The day after he returned to our new home in Colorado, Dick was out on the front deck, brushing Cliff. He called out for me to join him.

"Come and look at Cliff's back end and tail," Dick said. "I don't think it's laying the way it should." I could hear the concern in his voice.

"I haven't noticed anything strange, and I've been brushing them both every day," I said. While I had noticed that Cliff had been shedding a lot lately, I had attributed it to the change in altitude and climate. Dick had a strange look on his face.

"I think we should have this checked by a vet," he said. He asked me to call and get Cliff an appointment.

We didn't yet have a vet in Colorado, as Cliff and Jokonita had been getting their regular checkups in Pennsylvania. I opened up the phone book and found the listing for Steve's Dog & Cat Repair in Edwards, Colorado. I had driven past this clinic many times, and had always chuckled at the name. I had decided that when our dogs needed a vet, this would be where I would take them. I called and got an appointment for later that same afternoon.

When we arrived, a young female vet examined Cliff, checking his vitals and ordering some X-rays. After a few moments, she said, "I'm concerned that there's a tumor growing in his back end." Of course, I didn't think that was the case, and shrugged off any serious thought of it.

Shortly after the X-rays were taken, we were introduced to Dr. Stephen Warren, who told us that the films showed an abnormal mass growing on the right side of Cliff's anal area. Hearing this, I was in total disbelief. *How could this be?* Cliff was healthy, happy, and full of life. Dr. Warren talked about doing surgery to determine whether we were dealing with cancer. "I'd also like to draw some blood and do a CBC (complete blood count) and chemistry, to get a full understanding of Cliff's condition." Dr. Warren said.

"We'll do whatever's necessary, Doctor," I said, my voice sounding like it was coming from a tunnel. This all felt like a bad dream.

The blood work showed that Cliff had an abnormal white blood cell count, which meant there was an infection. Dr. Warren suggested that he put Cliff on an antibiotic drip immediately, to get the infection under control. Although this was the first time we had ever met Dr. Warren, both Dick and I felt totally comfortable with him, and confident about his decisions.

"I can do the surgery first thing tomorrow morning," Dr. Warren said, "but you'll have to leave Cliff here overnight."

That thought alone was hard enough for me to deal with; my happy days in the mountains were not supposed to involve leaving Cliff at a veterinary clinic overnight. But I knew it was the best thing for Cliff, so I bit my lip and tried to hold back the tears as I said good-bye and walked out the door.

On the way back to the house, I broke down. I couldn't keep my emotions in check any longer, and over the next several hours I was very quiet, the total opposite of my usual self. I was in shock—scared to death. Dick's happy Colorado homecoming had turned into a nightmare. Dick tried to comfort me, but both of us were at a loss for words. After a while, Dick told me that he felt guilty for not noticing the tumor sooner.

"There's no way we could've known," I said. "From the outside, Cliff appeared to be totally healthy. Just this morning, he was running around with Jokonita," I said, still in disbelief that this was actually happening.

Later that evening we got a phone call from a nurse at Dr. Warren's office. She told me that Cliff was resting comfortably with the IV drip, and that she'd call us in the morning to let us know how the surgery went.

Neither Dick nor I got much sleep that night.

The call came at 10:00 the next morning.

"Cliff is awake from the anesthesia," Dr. Warren said. "He's doing well, and you can come and pick him up."

With hardly a word, we rushed out the door and loaded Jokonita in the car. When we arrived at the clinic, I could tell by the look on Dr. Warren's face that the news was not good.

"I removed a mass from Cliff's anal gland," he said. "It was encapsulated, about the size of an egg." *Encapsulated* meant that it was self-contained, or confined to a specific area.

With my lack of knowledge about cancer, I was optimistic that he had removed it all. Dr. Warren told us that he'd sent half of the mass to IDEXX, a veterinary services lab in Denver, for a biopsy, and that he would have the results in a few days. He offered to show us the rest of the mass, but we declined. That was a picture I preferred not to carry around with me for the rest of my life.

When Dr. Warren brought him out to us, Cliff looked the same as he had the day before, except that his back leg had been shaved extensively at the site of the surgery, and he had stitches. Cliff bounded over, so happy to see us; you never would have known he'd just had surgery. He didn't seem a bit worried about his shaved leg. I went over to him, kneeling down to hug him.

"Everything's going to be okay," I whispered in Cliff's ear. "You're coming home with your Momma now." He seemed to understand, and quietly followed us out to the car.

We were sent home with some antibiotics, and told that they would call us when the results of the biopsy came in. Dr. Warren had prescribed a course of treatment for Cliff that included another ten days on the antibiotics and a warm compress applied to the surgical site a few times a day, to keep it clean. I was told to keep Cliff's activity level to a minimum for a few days to make sure the stitches did not pull loose; as long as the stitches stayed intact, the incision should heal well on its own. I was not very happy about how much of Cliff's leg had been shaved, but as Dick reminded me, that was the least of our worries.

The next few days passed in a blur. We tried to maintain our normal routine, and even though we had to somewhat restrict Cliff's activity level, we still took short hikes. I took extra time to sit with Cliff and Nita at my favorite overlook, thankful for this quiet time with them. I snuggled close to both dogs, contemplating all that may lie ahead of us. What if this was cancer? What would that mean for Cliff?

What would that mean for all of us?

5
The Diagnosis

The discovery of Cliff's tumor had changed everything. It definitely dampened my enthusiasm over my upcoming birthday on August 30, but I tried to go through the motions and appear happy. My fortieth birthday was one that I had been anticipating for a long while, a landmark in my life I was happy to have achieved. The fact that my mother had died in her mid-forties was always close at hand when my birthday came around, and even more so this year. I made Dick promise not to tell me if the phone call came on the thirtieth. I did not want to remember this as the day we'd found out Cliff had cancer. Although Dick kept his promise, he did receive the call that day. I knew it, and suspected what the results of the biopsy would reveal.

That night, we went to dinner at the Golden Eagle in Beaver Creek. Our group included Dick and me, my sister Amy and her husband Andy, their four-month-old son Chase, and some close friends of ours from the valley. Up to that point, I hadn't discussed my fears about Cliff with them, and I avoided talking about it during dinner. I think I was still very much in denial. I tried my best to have a good time and participate in the conversation and laughter, but all the while, I could not get Cliff out of my mind.

The following day we met with Dr. Warren, and he gave us a copy of the biopsy from IDEXX. The diagnosis was not good.

Source/History:
Mass, right anal gland region

Diagnosis:
Adenocarcinoma, apocrine gland/anal sac origin,
moderately differentiated

Comments:
Neoplastic cells extend to the specimen margin. There
is a high potential for local recurrence and progression.
There is moderate to high potential for regional and
systemic metastasis. Metastasis, when it occurs, is typically
to regional lymph nodes (sub-lumbar, etc.), and then to
the lungs and other body systems.

This neoplasm is often associated with humoral hyper-
calcemia of malignancy.

No evidence of vascular tumor embolization was found
in the sections examined.

I didn't understand all of this medical jargon, and as a result, did not realize how bad it truly was. The only good news we were given was that Cliff's chest X-rays were clear; the cancer had not spread to his lungs. They were still uncertain about whether there was any progression into the lymph nodes, and further tests would need to be done to determine this.

As we discussed our options, Dr. Warren told us that Colorado State University had a great veterinary teaching hospital and a cancer research center. Dick and I were not exactly sure what to do next, but since we planned to return to Pennsylvania in two days, we decided to meet with our vet there to see what treatment options he recommended for Cliff.

We returned to Pennsylvania, and on September 7, I took Cliff in to see our vet, Dr. Alan Friedlander, in State College. I explained to him what had been found, and that Dr. Warren had removed the tumor. I also gave him a copy of the blood work and biopsy. After examining Cliff, Dr. Friedlander decided to do more X-rays on his chest and lungs to make sure the cancer had not spread.

While talking with Dr. Friedlander, I met a young woman vet I hadn't met before—Dr. Debra Smart. She took an immediate interest in us, and told me that she was a graduate of the Colorado State University Veterinary Teaching Hospital (CSU VTH). At the time, this didn't mean much to me; I knew very little about the Veterinary Teaching Hospital, and I was also distracted by the stark realities of Cliff's diagnosis.

We talked briefly, and I told her about our new home in Colorado, and about Dr. Warren's recommendation. She agreed with Dr. Warren, and explained that the VTH had a very highly respected oncology department. She was very direct and confident when I asked for her opinion on treatment options for Cliff.

"If you're able to have him treated at CSU, then you should go there as soon as possible. The fact that you have a home three hours away from the VTH is an added bonus," Dr. Smart said. "In my opinion, Cliff will have the best chance of fighting the cancer if he is treated there."

That was all I needed to hear. I decided to go back to Colorado as soon as possible. Dr. Smart gave me the phone number for the CSU VTH, recommending that I try to get an appointment to see Dr. Stephen Withrow. "He's the head of surgery and oncology, and one of the best animal oncologists in the world," she said with a reassuring smile.

With the number in hand, I went home and told Dick that Cliff, Jokonita, and I would be returning to Colorado in three days. I was scared to death. I had no idea what I was getting myself or Cliff into; I just knew that I was trusting the referral of someone who, even though I didn't know her well, was totally, without a doubt, convinced that this was where we should go.

On Saturday, September 9, Penn State was playing at home. I went to the tailgate party in the morning, but explained to my friends and family that I would not be attending the game because I had to go home and pack. I'd be leaving for Colorado the next day. The weekend was filled with many emotions, and fear of the unknown topped the list. Dick offered to keep Jokonita in Pennsylvania with him while I took Cliff to Colorado, but I said no. I felt in my heart that it would be best for the three of us to go together, and Dick was totally supportive of my decision.

6
Saving Cliff

On Sunday morning, September 10, I headed to the airport with Cliff and Jokonita, not knowing when I would return to Pennsylvania, to my family, my friends, and my life there.

When I woke up in my Colorado home on Monday morning, the first thing I did was call the CSU Veterinary Teaching Hospital. I spoke to a woman at the appointment desk, explaining our situation, and asked for an appointment as soon as possible with Dr. Stephen Withrow. Fortunately for us, he had an opening, and I was told to come in the next day.

I had no idea where I was going, or how long I was going to be there, but I knew we would need a place to stay, for a few days at least. I called the hospital again, and asked if they knew of a hotel where I could stay with the dogs. The receptionist gave me the number for the Holiday Inn, and I called right away to make a reservation. We had to be at the CSU VTH on Tuesday at 9:30 A.M., so on Monday afternoon I loaded up the Suburban with Cliff, Jokonita, and my road bike. Unsure of how long we would be gone, I was prepared to stay as long as necessary.

This would be my first trip to Fort Collins, where the CSU VTH was located, and I was not exactly sure how long the drive would take. It ended up taking just a little under three hours, but then I still had to twist and turn from one unfamiliar street to another to find the hotel. I pulled into the parking lot and decided to check in before I let Cliff and Jokonita out of the Suburban. I asked for a room on one of the lower floors, but was told that all they had at the moment were rooms on the fourth floor or higher. I knew that going up and down on an elevator in

29

the middle of the night with two large dogs was not exactly ideal, but with no other options available, I took a room on the fourth floor, near the elevator.

I went back out to the car, opened the door, and both Cliff and Jokonita jumped out. I put their leashes on and walked them around on the grass. Frightened and worried about what lay ahead of us the next day, I was running on autopilot. I had never before stayed in a hotel with them. I wasn't sure how it was going to go, especially the late-night walks. It was fortunate for me that they were well-mannered and did whatever I asked of them—even Jokonita, who now followed along and behaved as well as Cliff did.

I think the first ride up in the elevator was a little unnerving for them, especially because the elevator had a glass front that looked out over the lobby. We got on, and when I pushed the button for it to start, they both seemed a little perplexed, giving me a wide-eyed look. As the elevator began to move, they sat down as if to steady themselves. I bent down and put my arms around them, to reassure them that everything was okay.

We got to our room, and I found that I was wiped out from the drive. I felt nauseous and my body was quivering. I ordered room service and a bottle of wine, and fed Cliff and Jokonita the Boston Market rotisserie turkey I'd bought on the way. Together, we settled in for our first evening in Fort Collins. Around 9:00 P.M. we made our first trip down the elevator, and I was relieved that things were actually going pretty smoothly. When we got to the lobby, the door of the elevator opened; standing there waiting to get in was a middle-aged couple. I looked at them and quickly assured them that Cliff and Jokonita were friendly. They took a step back to allow us to exit, and I smiled at them.

We returned to our room a little while later, and although I tried to settle down, sleep proved to be elusive. The wine had taken the edge off, but I was still very jittery and uneasy about our appointment the next day.

I woke very early the following morning, knowing that Cliff and Jokonita would need some exercise before we went to our appointment. I had no idea where I could take them to run, but I grabbed a canvas bag and put a couple of Frisbees in it, just to be prepared. I hooked them to their leashes, and we headed out the door on the side of the hotel, where I'd noticed an empty lot. I unleashed them both and threw the Frisbees. We played for about half an hour before going back to the hotel so I could take a quick shower.

I was a little anxious about leaving Jokonita alone for the first time in a hotel room. I knew she wouldn't be destructive, but still worried that she might bark, not understanding why Cliff and I had left her behind. I decided to give it a try, and left the television on to keep her company.

I took Cliff down and put him in the Suburban, then ran back up to check on Jokonita. I walked up to the door to listen, and even though I didn't hear anything, I felt like I needed to see her again, to reassure her that I would be coming back. As I inserted my key, she heard me and barked. I went inside and sat with her for a minute, telling her again that it would be all right; that I was just taking Cliff to his appointment, and would be back soon. I left again, and this time I stopped partway down the hall to find out whether she would start to bark. She didn't, making me feel a little more comfortable about leaving her alone. I'd made sure to leave the DO NOT DISTURB sign on the door handle so she would not be surprised by the housekeeping staff.

When I got back to the car, I told Cliff that we were going to see another doctor, one who I hoped would be able to help us. Cliff looked at me with his usual loving confidence, and I kissed the top of his head. I felt better than I had the day before; I was doing something concrete to help Cliff.

The drive from the hotel took less than five minutes, and as I pulled into the parking lot, I felt very strong and composed. I was determined that we were going to get through this. I opened up the back of the

Suburban, and Cliff jumped out. We were a little early, so I let him walk around in the grass for a few minutes to explore and relieve himself before heading inside. When we walked in, I saw four women sitting at desks behind a long counter, underneath signs that indicated where to check in for various treatments. I walked over to the oncology desk and signed in.

"Please have a seat," the receptionist said kindly. "One of our senior veterinary students will be coming out to talk with you shortly." I thanked her and took a seat, Cliff sitting on the floor next to me. The room was filled with other people and their dogs, but I was oblivious to them all. I just sat there with Cliff, rubbing his head and talking to him, trying to stay calm and in control. A short while later, a young female veterinary student approached us.

"Hi—I'm Tara. Is this Cliff?" she asked, with a smile.

"Yes," I said.

As she bent down to pet Cliff, she spoke calmly to him, and I felt a sense of ease. Tara asked me to follow her into one of the exam rooms, which featured a large metal table with an adjustable light hanging overhead. Along the back wall was a sink with some cabinets above and below it. I noticed a long wooden bench, and I took a seat on it while Cliff sat next to me on the floor. Tara had a form with her, and asked me some questions regarding Cliff's medical history. When we'd finished filling out the form, she left, telling me that Dr. Withrow would be in to see us soon.

A short time later, Dr. Withrow came in. He looked to be in his fifties, partly graying and very distinguished-looking. With him was a woman he introduced as Dr. Kim Selting. She was slender and had long, dark brown hair; the minute she smiled at me, I felt an instant connection. I turned to listen to Dr. Withrow as he talked about cancer, and the various options we had available to us. He said that he had reviewed the X-rays that I had brought along, along with the biopsy report.

"I think we should do another surgery—go in and get any cancer that may still be there, to try to get clean margins," Dr. Withrow said. "I'd also like to do an ultrasound to see if Cliff's lymph nodes are enlarged, and to see how Cliff's testicles and prostate look." He also ordered another CBC and some chest X-rays to make sure his lungs were still clean.

I soon found out that if "narrow margins" are found, a second surgery is often performed in an attempt to obtain "clean margins." When cancer spreads to other organs, it may or may not have made it out of the primary tumor successfully prior to that tumor's removal; it's hard to know for certain. So, when the doctors look at the tissue under the microscope and see that the tumor cells are very near the normal tissue margins (meaning, where the surgical blade went), they are concerned that another section might show that they go to the edge (meaning, some cells may have been left behind that could grow back).

Despite feeling a bit overwhelmed by all of this information, my first impression of Dr. Withrow was a positive one. Here was someone I could trust completely. He answered the many questions I had in a direct fashion, and while I sensed he had heard the same questions many times before, he still took the time to fully explain his answers. I felt like he had the situation under control, and that I wouldn't hesitate to do whatever it was he suggested.

"We're going to take Cliff for a while now, to have his blood drawn, and to schedule him for the ultrasound and X-rays," said Dr. Withrow. "You can either wait here, or leave and come back in a few hours for the results."

"I guess I'll go back and check on Jokonita at the hotel," I said.

"Good-bye, Cliff . . ." I whispered in his ear. "I'll be back soon. You'll be fine here." Cliff looked up at me, and I sensed he understood what I was saying. I was still very composed, for I felt like I was leaving Cliff in good hands.

When I got back to the hotel room, I was happy to see that Jokonita was fine. I decided to take her out for a while to play. Having her there with me helped take my mind off what was going on, and I was glad I'd brought her along.

After a few hours I returned to the VTH, checked in, and asked to have Dr. Withrow paged. We talked, and he told me that Cliff's CBC was fine, and that his ultrasound and X-rays looked good. There was no sign of the cancer spreading to his lymph nodes, prostate, testicles, or lungs. "We've scheduled the surgery for the next day, and we'll know more after that," he said.

Smiling, I said, "Thank you so much, Doctor."

Tara brought Cliff out to me, and the joy of our reunion far outweighed the fear I'd been experiencing. Before I left, Dr. Withrow asked me to have Cliff back at 7:30 the next morning for surgery. I was instructed not to give him any food or water after his evening meal. I nodded, and hurried out the door. I was so glad to get out of there!

I rushed back to the hotel to get Jokonita. I knew we wouldn't be spending the rest of the day in our room. I ended up driving through town until I saw a sign for Boyd Lake. I followed the signs to the lake, not knowing that this place would become our retreat during our days in Fort Collins. It was the perfect escape for us, fairly deserted in September, with lots of space to run. We spent the rest of the afternoon there playing Frisbee, walking along the shoreline, and enjoying the late-afternoon sunshine. We returned to the hotel in time to settle in for the evening. I wanted Cliff to get a good night's rest.

The next morning when I left the hotel with Cliff, I was not so worried about leaving Jokonita. I knew she had figured out that I would be coming back for her. I arrived at the VTH and was met by Tara. She talked to me about what would be happening that day, and said she needed to take Cliff back to get him ready for surgery.

"I'm going back to the hotel to get Jokonita and take her out for a walk," I said. I gave her my cell phone number and asked her to call me if she needed me.

"Will do," Tara said.

After a few hours in the park with Jokonita, I returned to the VTH. When I saw Dr. Withrow, he again had Dr. Selting with him.

"The surgery went well. We'll have the results back from the lab tomorrow," Dr. Withrow said. "Cliff is recovering nicely, but we'd like to keep him overnight for observation."

Hearing this, my heart sank. I knew I had no choice, but that didn't make it any easier. I was able to see him before I left, and knew I'd never forget the look in his eyes. He was wearing an Elizabethan collar—a big, white, plastic lampshade–type contraption that surrounded his entire head. They had put it on to prevent him from licking his incision, but I'm sure Cliff didn't understand that. He looked confused and sad, like he was wondering why he had this thing around his neck. I could hardly bear to see him like this, and tears filled my eyes as I sat with him, gently stroking his head.

"I've got to leave soon," I told him, "but I'll bring back some turkey for your dinner. You need to stay here tonight so they can keep an eye on you." I kissed his forehead and told him I would be back first thing in the morning to take him home.

I couldn't speak to anyone as I departed the building, and avoided looking at the staff members. When I got outside, I finally lost it. What had been building for the past few days came rushing out. I found a quiet spot under a tree and just sat there and cried. I no longer tried to fight it; I let it all out. I sat there for what seemed like hours, even though it was actually about thirty minutes. A sharp pain was shooting through my heart. I felt completely helpless and alone.

Once I'd regained my composure, I went back to the Suburban and was greeted with kisses from Jokonita. I wondered if she could taste the salt from my tears. Before heading to the hotel, I stopped at Boston Market again to pick up some turkey for Cliff. Although the food at the VTH was perfectly satisfactory, I felt that if I dropped off the turkey for them to feed Cliff, he would somehow know it came from me. Spoiling him with this treat had become a habit lately.

I hardly slept that night. I couldn't wait to get to the hospital to see Cliff the next morning.

When I returned to the VTH the next day, Dr. Withrow and Dr. Selting told me the margins were clear, but because they were so close to where the cancer had been, there was a possibility the cancer had metastasized to other areas.

"We recommend radiation therapy on the area around the surgery site, in case any cancer cells have already gotten through," Dr. Withrow said, "and we may want to do chemotherapy after that. In any case, we'd like to start the radiation as soon as the incision heals—most likely around the beginning of October."

"What does this mean, exactly?" I asked.

"Cliff will receive the radiation five days a week, for four weeks straight," Dr. Withrow explained.

I thought this sounded like a lot of radiation, and asked about it. I soon learned that different types of cancer require different amounts of radiation, generally anywhere from three to six weeks. For this particular type of cancer, four weeks would be the right amount.

"Will this affect Cliff's sperm?" I asked. "I'm still planning on breeding Cliff and Jokonita in the future." From the day I'd fallen in love with Cliff, I'd known that I wanted to raise his puppies. Cliff was unique; I felt it. This dog was a gentle giant who not only possessed a regal nature and a kind temperament, but also great intelligence and a strong male expression. He was the descendant of a world champion, and I felt that his qualities should be shared with future generations.

"We may be able to keep the testicles out of the radiation field," Dr. Selting said. "But first, we'll have to find out how wide the field needs to be."

"Can we bank some of Cliff's sperm before the treatment?" I asked.

"We don't do that here, but I can get you the name of someone who does offer that service," Dr. Selting said.

I smiled and thanked her.

"You can take Cliff home with you today," Dr. Selting continued. "You'll need to bring him back in a few weeks to have the stitches removed. And please be sure to keep the Elizabethan collar on him when he's not being closely watched, so that he doesn't lick or chew the stitches."

I nodded my assent. Once again, I felt suddenly overwhelmed to be facing so many unknowns.

Before we left, Dr. Withrow put his hand on my shoulder and wished me luck. I sensed that from that point on, it would be Dr. Selting who would be seeing us on a regular basis, and I was fine with that.

Dr. Selting and I talked for a while longer, as I had more questions for her.

"How exactly does radiation help?" I said. Obviously, I had heard of radiation therapy before, but I didn't really understand how it worked.

"Radiation is a specific type of energy that is generated by a special machine," Dr. Selting said. "A beam of this energy is delivered to the sites where the cancer cells are located. The radiation damages the cancer cells, which prevents them from growing and dividing. Once the cancer cells are damaged, they cannot repair themselves, and eventually—hopefully—all the cancer cells are destroyed," she concluded.

Hearing this gave me great hope that the radiation could rid Cliff of cancer.

Before leaving, Dr. Selting said that she would schedule Cliff's radiation to start the first week of October. "You'll need to have him at the VTH

CLIFF AND I

every morning at seven-thirty sharp," she said. "Check in with me in a few days, to let me know how Cliff is doing."

"Thanks for everything, Doctor. I'll stay in touch," I said.

I couldn't get out of the hospital fast enough, but despite everything, I left with an optimistic smile on my face. I had every confidence in Dr. Selting, and felt that the VTH was the right place for us to be.

Cliff and I walked across the parking lot to our car, and I loaded him in. As for the Elizabethan collar that Cliff was supposed to wear—I took it off as soon as I got him in the Suburban. I could tell that he didn't like wearing it, and I was not going to force him. I knew Cliff well enough to know he wouldn't mess with the stitches. He hadn't tried to pull them out after the first surgery, and I knew he wouldn't do it this time, either.

We went directly to the hotel, where I packed up our belongings. With both dogs safely in the back of the car, we were soon headed home to the mountains.

38

7
Banking Cliff's Sperm

SEPTEMBER 2000

The weekend back in the mountains was a quiet one for the three of us, and for the most part, Cliff did just fine, and seemed happy to be home.

The doctors had prescribed a variety of different medicines: two antibiotics, cephalexin and metronidazole, to fight infection; morphine for pain; and carprofen for the swelling. They had instructed me to keep an eye on Cliff's stitches, and to be sure they were kept clean. The doctors had given me a list of things to watch for that would indicate there might be a problem. If I noticed that the incision was swelling, or if it got really red, seemed tender, or started to ooze, I was to call the hospital right away. Also, if Cliff seemed to be in pain when he was relieving himself, or if he lost control when he had to go, I was to call the hospital. Dr. Selting had recommended a stool softener, since that area would probably be painful for a little while.

Before I'd left the hospital, Dr. Selting had given me the name of a person in Colorado Springs to contact regarding the banking of Cliff's sperm. In addition, she had said that the question of breeding a dog who had cancer had been brought up to her in the past. While many cancers have a heritable component, she noted, this particular type of cancer did not. Hearing this news made me feel comfortable about moving forward with my plans.

I made the call on Monday morning, only to be told that the doctor I was looking for was on sabbatical for a year, and that no one else at the clinic was doing sperm collection. The woman I spoke to gave me the name of someone else to call, at the Brighton Animal Clinic.

I called the Brighton clinic and explained that I wanted to bank the sperm of an eight-year-old German shepherd who had cancer, and was soon to undergo radiation and chemotherapy. The woman on the phone asked if I had a bitch—a female dog—to use as a teaser. Fortunately, Jokonita was just coming into heat. The woman gave us an appointment for the following week, telling me to bring both dogs with me. I didn't know where Brighton was located, but quickly discovered that it's just slightly northeast of Denver. I had no idea what to expect, but it sounded like this clinic performed a lot of these procedures. I decided to trust that they knew what they were doing.

I was very anxious on the morning of our appointment, and we left the house with plenty of time to spare. By now, Cliff had almost totally recovered from the surgery, and although he still had the stitches, he was pretty much back to his normal self—and very interested in Jokonita's condition.

I found the clinic without a problem, and once inside, I told the woman behind the counter my name and our appointment time. The waiting area was empty, so I took a seat along the back wall, Cliff and Jokonita sitting down next to me. A few minutes later, I was instructed to take them into the room next door. There were two people in the room: Dr. Sheri Beattie and a male technician named Jake, who I assumed was there to assist with the procedure.

At this point, I was very curious to see how the collection would actually take place, and at the same time, somewhat in awe of what was about to happen. I was told to give Jokonita's leash to Jake, who would hold her during the procedure. My job was to hold Cliff's head right behind Jokonita's back end. The doctor would do the rest.

I noticed then that Dr. Beattie had a funnel-type object in her hand in which she would collect the specimen. The actual collection took only a few minutes, and as soon as it was completed, Jake took Jokonita into a different room. I was told to take Cliff outside and let him walk it off.

Soon one of the technicians came outside and told me that she needed to take a DNA sample from Cliff. (I later learned that as of October 1, 1998, the American Kennel Club [AKC] requires that any dog whose semen is frozen for storage, or collected and used as fresh semen, must have a DNA profile on record at the AKC.) As I held Cliff's mouth open, she scraped inside with a toothbrush-type object. The sample would be analyzed, and the results sent to me. She asked that I forward a copy to their office when I received it.

I was amazed at this point. Not only had I just learned how sperm was collected, but I'd also learned that they now take DNA samples from dogs. I assured her that when I got the report, I'd get a copy to them. With that completed, I loaded Cliff in the Suburban and went back inside to get Jokonita.

Once inside, I was told the semen evaluation was just about finished, and I could wait for a copy of it. A few minutes later, Dr. Beattie came out to explain the results. "We collected enough sperm for eighteen inseminations," she said. "Most people keep enough for five or six, but it's up to you to decide what you'd like to do."

"Keep them all," I said, without hesitation. I knew that I wanted to have as many chances as possible for a successful insemination.

"That won't be a problem," Dr. Beattie said. "The samples will be divided for individual use."

She went on to explain the semen evaluation form, which showed that it was a very good collection. Only 4 percent were bent, and out of the total collection, 30 percent were abnormal and 70 percent were normal. Although I had no prior knowledge of this procedure, I felt very positive about the collection, and glad that I'd had it done.

Dr. Beattie explained how to access the semen when needed, and told me that I would have to fill out a release form before the semen could be shipped. *Wow, this is serious business,* I thought. Nonetheless, I felt reassured that the process had been handled in such a professional manner.

I thanked them all for their assistance, and said that I'd be in touch to let them know how things were going with us. Before I left, I was given a packet that included information on shipping, and some release forms. I also found a bumper sticker that read MY DOG BANKS WITH ICSB, FIRST IN FROZEN ASSETS, INTERNATIONAL CANINE SEMEN BANK—COLORADO. I chuckled and thought, How appropriate.

On the drive home that afternoon, I kept a close eye on Cliff to see how he was doing. He seemed very interested in Nita, who was at the point in her cycle at which she was receptive to his advances. I continued to keep them apart, however, since I didn't think the timing was right for her to get pregnant. We had a long battle ahead of us with Cliff's upcoming radiation treatments.

And chemotherapy was still a dark possibility lurking in our future.

8
Radiation Therapy

Our first week of radiation completed, we were headed back to the mountains for a few days of rest. I was feeling pretty good. For the most part, Cliff had handled the daily treatments very well, and so far, he'd shown no outward signs of the radiation, except for the shaved area on his right leg and rear end, and the X marks at the treatment site. I knew it would be good for us to have a few days of downtime to enjoy the mountains. Plus, Dick would be returning to Colorado the next day, giving me some much-needed emotional support.

It had been a long month on my own. Even though I'd constantly drawn on the strength in Cliff's eyes—he'd been such a trooper during each treatment—it would be good to have a human shoulder, too. Before we left town, I decided to stop at the Boston Market to pick up dinner for Cliff and Jokonita. I already had the Suburban packed and ready to go, so as soon as I picked Cliff up from the VTH, I would head to Boyd Lake to feed them and let them play a little before we started our drive home.

We had been going to Boyd Lake every day after Cliff's radiation treatments. Sometimes we played Frisbee, and sometimes we just walked along the shoreline while I looked for trinkets in the sand, filling my pockets with interesting bottle caps or small, rounded stones. When it was hot, I usually let the dogs get in the water to cool off, but I knew that those days would be ending soon. Once Cliff's radiation spots started to get raw, he wouldn't be able to go in the water and risk the chance of picking up an infection.

As I pulled into our usual lot, close to a grassy area and a picnic pavilion, I saw only a few boats on the water. Once again, I felt thankful that this place had been so deserted during the times we'd visited. Two heads shot up from the back of the Suburban; the dogs were excited to see where we were, and ready to play. I opened the back door and out they jumped, their Frisbees clamped in their mouths. I looked at Cliff, and felt thankful that he had tolerated the radiation so well this past week. I only hoped that the next three weeks would go as smoothly.

I started to pull the turkey apart, putting it in their bowls to let it cool off. I could tell Cliff was anxious to eat, and felt grateful that he hadn't lost his appetite. Although I knew I was spoiling them with this special treat—something both dogs had gotten used to during our trips to Fort Collins—in reality, the turkey was a very convenient source of the protein Cliff needed right now. Soon after Cliff's diagnosis, I had learned about the importance of proper nutrition in his fight against cancer. I often heard the phrase, "Feed the patient, starve the tumor." Research indicated that a diet high in protein and low in carbohydrates would do just that. I felt the extra turkey I gave Cliff could only help, as it was a great source of lean protein—not to mention the fact that he loved it and ate it willingly.

It was later on that I learned of a specially formulated pet food that was designed with the cancer patient in mind: Hill's Pet Nutrition—Prescription Diet Canine n/d. This food fulfills the dog's caloric requirements, and has the correct balance of protein, carbohydrates, and fats.

When the dogs had finished their meal, I rinsed out their bowls and gave them some water. I didn't plan to spend a lot of time at the lake today, as I wanted to head back to the mountains. I looked around, and seeing no one on the beach, I grabbed my bag and told them to get their Frisbees. I felt happy to be with them, sharing this special part of our daily routine.

We walked along the shoreline, and as I glanced down, I noticed their paw prints in the sand. I quickly pulled out my camera and snapped some pictures of the prints. I could easily tell which ones were Cliff's, as his feet were much larger than Jokonita's. I wasn't exactly sure why I'd felt the urge to take the pictures; maybe because I wanted to capture every moment of the times we were sharing together. These pictures would help to remind me of all we had gone through, and of all the places we had been. I glanced up from the sand to see both of them standing there, looking at me as if to say, *Come on, Mom—let's play!*

We continued down to the water's edge, where I threw the Frisbee for them to chase. Once we got that close to the water, they would usually go in before I could give them permission. Jokonita dropped her Frisbee as she took a drink of water, biting at the water instead of licking at it. I quickly stepped in to grab the Frisbee before it sank or floated away. The two dogs romped for a while, splashing and biting at the water. I still had my camera out, so I snapped a few more shots. I glanced at my watch and realized that in order to avoid the Denver rush hour, we needed to dry off and get back on the road. I called for them both to come out of the water, and we headed back to the parking lot.

Along the way I stopped under a tree and took some more pictures of them. I couldn't help myself. Cliff was so handsome, standing very much at attention, his eyes staring intensely at me. I looked into those eyes, and saw in them the affection that we shared. I smiled to myself, feeling so grateful for that gift of love. My initial plan was to focus on a head-and-shoulder shot of him, as a big part of me didn't want to see the shaved leg and radiation X's. But I suddenly realized that those X's were a symbol of what we were going through. Even if they were not captured in the photos, there was no denying that they were there.

So, after hesitating for a moment, I took some full-body shots of Cliff, with the radiation X's in full sight. Maybe these very battle scars would help us both hang on, serving as a reminder of how much we had lived through to get to this point. They would also signify how much more still lay ahead of us . . . the many unknowns yet to face. Would I be able to draw strength from these pictures at the times I'd need it the most? Yes, I thought—I could. If Cliff could undergo the treatments and still maintain his zest for life, I was determined to be right by his side with the same level of commitment.

As we returned to the Suburban, the dogs ran ahead. I was glad to see that Cliff still looked as agile as ever. I knew we still had many battles left to fight, but I was feeling very good about the care he was receiving at the VTH. I knew that I had made the right choice in coming to Colorado, and was grateful to be here with him. I knew that if we could get through the next few weeks, there would be many happy days ahead for us.

I felt confident that I was strong enough to see this through; I just hoped and prayed that Cliff had enough trust in me. I also hoped he would understand, even when the treatments got harder on him, that I was doing this for him because I loved him, and because it provided his best chance for recovery. Even though I hadn't known them for very long, I had total confidence in Dr. Selting and the staff at the VTH. This was where we needed to be.

I grabbed some towels out of the car and bent down to wipe the dogs, only to find that they were nearly dry; I just needed to wipe off their feet and bellies. I opened up the back doors of the car, and they simultaneously jumped in. I was happy to see that Cliff could still do that. I told them that we were going back to the mountains, and would be home in a couple of hours. I was glad it wasn't winter yet, because I didn't look forward to climbing these mountain highways in snowy or icy conditions. I dreaded the thought of anything getting in the way of taking Cliff to his treatments.

I looked in my rearview mirror and saw that they were both lying down and resting comfortably. I decided to pop in a CD and get "in the zone." The drive home had become a form of therapy for me, allowing me time to work things out in my mind—to process all the conflicting emotions that filled my days, and absorb all that the doctors had told me.

I really felt that this reflection time helped me to make clear decisions about Cliff's care.

A little less than three hours later, I pulled into our garage. Cliff and Jokonita began to wag their tails and move around in the back. They looked eager to get out, and happy to be home. So was I. Once released, Cliff ran over to the closest tree to leave his mark. *It's good to see that some things never change,* I thought, smiling.

I went into the house to see if there were any messages on the answering machine, and there were—but nothing that couldn't wait. I glanced out the kitchen window to see that Cliff and Jokonita were up on the hillside already, sitting and waiting for me to join them. How wonderful it felt to be back in the mountains! A walk in the fresh air would do us all a world of good. As we headed up the mountain, I heard the familiar sound of the squirrels. By the look of Cliff's and Jokonita's quivering ears, they had, too. We walked into the forest, and I inhaled the scent of the earth, feeling blessed. These quiet moments of peace would sustain me in the weeks and months to come.

I watched them as they romped a few feet in front of me, now running from tree to tree, chasing a squirrel. It was lucky for the creature that neither Cliff nor Jokonita had mastered the art of tree climbing yet! I allowed them the freedom to chase squirrels in this safe place, one where Jokonita was more likely to stay close. The dogs welcomed the chance to play one of their favorite games. In a short while, we were pretty far up the mountain, and the sun was starting to set. I called them to join me for our walk back to the house. On the way, I passed a large aspen tree where unbeknownst to me, Dick had carved Cliff's name into the trunk shortly after Cliff's diagnosis. I wouldn't realize until years later how important this tree would become to me.

I spent the rest of the evening on the sofa, sipping wine and watching TV, with my two "kids" on either side of me, relaxed and happy to be home. Even though we hadn't lived here very long, this was definitely the place I called home—the place I felt most at peace. I was glad we had this refuge to come to, especially now, during Cliff's treatment.

Later that night while lying in bed, my head was just inches away from Cliff's as he rested his head on the pillow next to me. I looked into his eyes, staring into mine. His eyes often reflected a wide range of emotions—excitement, curiosity, joy, fear. I could often interpret his feelings from even a subtle shift in his eyes. I tried to read them now. *What are you thinking, Cliff?* These last few weeks had been challenging. *Does he understand why we are here?*

As I silently pondered this, I sensed that somehow, he *did* understand. I leaned over and kissed the very top of his nose, and smiled. These quiet moments we shared transcended the need for speech.

The next morning I told the dogs we were going to the airport to pick up Daddy. Dick was scheduled to arrive at 2:00 P.M., and as we drove through the gate at the private terminal, we could see that he'd already landed and was standing outside the plane. The minute the dogs saw him, they responded with excitement. I got out to greet Dick, letting Cliff and Jokonita out, too. They quickly ran over to him, tails wagging, their happiness at seeing him clearly evident. Dick was equally pleased to be reunited with all of us.

On the ride home, I filled Dick in on the details of our week.

"I think Cliff is doing really well with the radiation," I said. "I just hope it'll keep going this smoothly."

"I'm sure it will," Dick said confidently. He was as impressed as I was with the quality of care Cliff had been receiving at the VTH—and like me, he believed in Cliff's strength.

The next morning we awakened to clear blue skies—the kind of day that takes your breath away. I decided that after I took Cliff and Jokonita out for a walk on the mountain, I would head out on my bike for a few hours. I felt the need to burn off some energy, and knew that a ride would do me good. Having Dick there made me feel better about leaving Cliff and Jokonita for a while.

When I returned from my ride, I entered the house through the garage. I had expected to see Cliff and Jokonita running to greet me, but they weren't there. I didn't even hear them. I noticed that the 4Runner was still there, so I assumed that Dick was out on the mountain with them.

I ran upstairs to the loft to do a quick check of e-mail, and as I sat down, I heard the back door open. I heard the sound of Nita and Cliff running in, and realized that Dick had been out back with the dogs, most likely brushing or playing with them. I started to tell Dick about my ride, but he stopped me.

"Cliff had a really bad case of diarrhea while you were gone," he said, sounding anxious.

As I stood there, looking down over the railing, I noticed two piles of vomit on the wood floor in the dining room. I looked at Dick. Although neither of us wanted to say it out loud, we both wondered if this was it—the moment we'd been dreading. Dr. Selting had said that the radiation would most likely cause side effects, and I was afraid that the moment had come. I realized again that we still had a long battle ahead of us.

Dr. Selting had given me some medicine for diarrhea and nausea in case we needed it, and I quickly went and found it. I gave it to Cliff and decided I would wait a little while before I fed him, so that it would have time to work. As the afternoon progressed, Cliff seemed more energetic, and acted like he was feeling better. When I did feed him later on, he ate all of his dinner and was able to keep it down. This gave me some hope that what he'd experienced that afternoon wasn't too serious—at least, not yet.

A few weeks later, we were back in Fort Collins to start Cliff's last week of radiation. The intervening weeks had gone smoothly. Cliff had tolerated the radiation well, and I'd kept him on the medicine for his stomach, which was working great—no more signs of nausea and diarrhea. I was very much looking forward to finishing this course of treatment, which meant no more daily trips to the VTH at 7:30 A.M. I was hoping some sense of normalcy would return to our lives.

But this day had started out differently than the past few mornings, with Cliff waking me at 5:00 to let me know he needed to go out. He had been on morphine for any pain he might have been experiencing at the radiation site. The mornings had become the most difficult for us, since he fought the urge to relieve himself because of the pain. Once the morphine kicked in, he was okay, but it was always a chore to get him to take the pill. (I usually tried to hide it in a piece of cheese, but he'd started to eye each piece suspiciously. Sometimes I thought he was just too smart for his own good!)

I could tell that his morphine had worn off on this particular morning, and he seemed very uncomfortable. The cheese hadn't worked well, so I'd found some leftover turkey in the fridge and I hid the tiny purple pill inside it. Finally, success! The morphine would soon be in his system, and he would get some relief from the pain. I was thankful that it would kick in by the time he went in for radiation.

We headed back to bed. I knew that if I lay back down, so would Cliff, and in an hour or so, he'd be feeling much better. Lying there, I wished Dick was still with me. He'd left a few days before, and now I faced the final days of Cliff's radiation treatment on my own. Dick had been a huge help, taking Cliff to the VTH on some mornings, which allowed me extra time with Jokonita. I was glad he'd spent some time in Fort Collins with us, and that he'd been able to meet Dr. Selting and some of her colleagues at the VTH. But now it was just the three of us again, and I knew that I needed to hang in there for a few more days.

Dr. Selting had underscored the importance of completing the entire cycle of radiation. We only had four more treatments after the session today. Cliff's rear end had now become raw and swollen, and I prayed that it would heal quickly.

Cliff and Jokonita were both lying next to me; I knew that we all found comfort in being so close together when we slept. Cliff had rarely slept in my bed before he got cancer, preferring his own cushy foam bed on the floor, next to mine—always protecting me, even when he slept. Now, he was the first one to jump on the bed and take his place next to me. As I lay there, watching the minutes tick away on the clock, I knew that I had to get up and get going soon. Cliff was more alert and moving around, so I was pretty sure the morphine had kicked in.

As we made our way to the VTH later that morning, the skies were gray, and a light rain was falling. David, one of the senior veterinary students, greeted us when we arrived. A tall man with blond hair and eyebrows, David had a huge heart; he'd shown us great compassion during the past week. It was nice to see his friendly, smiling face again.

"Hey, Cliff—how're you doing?" David asked, rubbing behind Cliff's ears.

I smiled, and thanked David for his kindness. I was glad that Cliff would be with him during his final week of radiation. David seemed to genuinely care about what we were going through, and I found a lot comfort in that. In fact, I'd come to realize that everyone we'd met at the VTH was thoughtful and compassionate. We were not just a number to them. We were so fortunate that this hospital was here, teaching these talented young men and women how to be great doctors, and how to care for our most beloved friends.

After a final hug, I turned Cliff over to David, knowing that Cliff understood I'd be back soon. I'd be sitting in the same chair, waiting for him to come running to meet me. Most days he'd be pulling whoever was on the other end of the leash in his haste to reach me. Every day when he came back to me, I could see the love and trust in his eyes.

I left the VTH and took Jokonita to the park to play. It was drizzling outside, but neither of us really minded the rain. As I stood there, a light mist falling all around me, I glanced up at the sky and noticed a break in the clouds. At first, I thought the break was just a tease, a "sucker hole," with no blue skies behind it. But this was no sucker hole. The clouds slowly dissipated, and the sky began to clear—in a very strange way. It did not clear everywhere, but only right above the spot where I was standing. I no longer felt alone. I felt very calm. I had an eerie feeling that some force was there with me.

I played with Jokonita for a while, and the longer I stood there, the clearer it became—not only the sky, but also my mind. *I had become a different person.* This experience had changed me a great deal. While I often felt sad facing cancer with Cliff, I also felt empowered. I'd discovered I could be strong when I needed to be. Often at night, I would call Dr. Selting, knowing full well that I would get her voice mail. At those times I would ramble on, expressing my fears and concerns. Much later, Dr. Selting told me she'd been happy to receive my late-night messages. She was relieved to know that I was letting it all out, understanding how vitally important it was for me to deal with my emotions as I was feeling them in order to avoid troubling times in the future.

I headed back to the hotel and got Jokonita settled in our room. Despite the chill, I changed into a pair of black cycling shorts and a short-sleeved jersey, grabbed my raincoat for the continuing drizzle, and set out on my bike toward the lake. Along the way, I had to cross a busy intersection, so I unclipped my feet from the pedals and waited for traffic to clear. As I stood there waiting, I saw an old green army truck stopped at the other side of the intersection. The paint on the truck was faded, and what appeared to have been a large red cross painted on the side had turned to mostly white. I carefully crossed the street and noticed that there was a driver in the truck, dressed in fatigues. As I followed the truck down the street, it reminded me of something from the *M*A*S*H* television series, years ago. I found it odd that I'd seen it at this moment.

I recognized the side street in front of me, and found the entrance to the bike path around the lake. My legs were numb from the cold air, and I realized that it was starting to rain harder. The droplets of rain were accumulating along the brim of my helmet, and I had to periodically shake my head to knock them off. I rode past the swim beach and noticed a first-aid station with a large red cross painted on it. *Why am I seeing red crosses today?* I wondered. *Was this a sign for me to be more careful?* The trail was now covered with wet leaves, so I slowed down.

I continued on the bike path, past Mussel Beach, and thought back to the last time I'd been there with Cliff. It had been a warm, sunny day, and several beautiful butterflies had fluttered all around us. The memory brought a smile to my face. I thought about Cliff, and I longed to return to that day. I headed back to the highway and passed a truck that read SHAMROCK FOODS; it had four-leaf clovers on it.

I started to connect the things I'd seen so far that day. A sudden clearing in the sky; red crosses; four-leaf clovers. Was it possible there was a message to me in all of these things? Was I going crazy? Was I imagining all of this? Why was I taking notice of these things today—things that most days I would ride right past and not think twice about?

Something had happened to me in the last few weeks. I felt different. I not only felt more connected to Cliff, but also to the entire world around me. I had developed a deeper appreciation for the simplest of things: the water rippling on the lake; the moon appearing in the sky; the rain gently falling on my face; the quiet times I spent with Cliff as we silently communicated with each other, his head resting on my lap. Living through these days with Cliff had forced me to slow down. This was the positive element of a situation that at times was extremely painful.

The next four days of radiation were the hardest on Cliff. It was worse than anything I could have anticipated. Cliff was agitated and had difficulty sleeping, in reality, neither one of us got much sleep. Although he was on morphine, he was still uncomfortable, and I often heard him whimpering. In addition, he had such severe gas that I often had to get up in the middle of the night to spray perfume in the room to mask the odor.

I discussed all of this with Dr. Selting, telling her that I just couldn't do it anymore—I wanted to stop the radiation. She was quick to reassure me.

"The last few days of radiation are not only the hardest on Cliff, but also the most critical, as he'll be receiving the most significant doses of radiation during these treatments," Dr. Selting said. "We've come this far—it's very important that we finish."

I had no idea when we'd started that after sixteen treatments, I would be ready to quit, with just four sessions to go. But I'd also had no idea of the amount of pain and discomfort that Cliff would experience during the final days. In comparison, the first three weeks had been relatively easy. Although I knew we couldn't quit, I also felt that I didn't know how to proceed. Was there anything that could help Cliff during this difficult phase?

Dr. Selting suggested that they increase the frequency of the oral morphine to every four to six hours, and also that they put a fentanyl patch (a morphine-like drug) on Cliff's leg to provide a continual low dose of the drug. I was thankful to find that the patch and the increase in the morphine helped significantly. I saw a change in Cliff right after the increase, and knew then that we could make it a few more days.

Soon after this discussion, Dr. Selting broke the news that Cliff would be receiving chemotherapy once his radiation treatments had been completed.

I was disheartened to hear this, but knew that I had to proceed with whatever they recommended. Dr. Selting assured me that most dogs tolerate chemo very well, and it does not seem to have the same adverse side effects on dogs as it does on humans. I was happy to hear that dogs do not lose their hair, as humans do. *If we can survive the radiation, we can survive the chemo,* I thought to myself.

On October 27, 2000, Cliff had his final radiation treatment. When he was brought out to me in the waiting room, he wore an orange handkerchief around his neck that read HAPPY HALLOWEEN, and HUG ME—I'VE HAD RADIATION THERAPY AT COLORADO STATE UNIVERSITY. I sat down next to Cliff and did just that, hugging him tightly.

"I'm so proud of you," I whispered in his ear. He had done his part; he'd been the model patient. We were given our dismissal papers and told to return on November 21 to begin the chemotherapy.

A week later, Cliff's morphine intake was reduced to only once every twelve hours, and he was off the morphine patch. He was still taking some anti-inflammatory drugs, and they seemed to be doing what they were supposed to do. My main concern was that he was still straining when he had to relieve himself, but at least he was no longer whimpering, and he didn't appear to be in any pain. His back end, where he'd received the largest doses of radiation, was still very red and irritated, but after a week, the sticky yellow discharge from the dead skin had cleared away.

I'd been cleaning the pungent, foul-smelling radiated area with povidone iodine, and the odor had disappeared. I would moisten a washcloth and squeeze a small amount of the povidone iodine on it, using my fingers to work it in until a yellow foam appeared. Then, as Cliff lay on the floor, I would sit next to him and gently raise his tail, pressing the cloth on the radiated area and holding it there for a few minutes. I could tell he wasn't crazy about me messing around in that area, so as I sat there, I would stroke his head and tell him that it was okay; I was just trying to make it feel better.

I then gently applied aloe and vitamin E to the area. I knew it must have caused a burning sensation, because Cliff would walk around in circles, trying to shake it off. He was a very smart dog, however, and when I told him not to lick the ointment, he listened. After a few minutes, he seemed to calm down, and lost interest in it.

Now that Cliff was beginning to heal, I was even more confident about the decisions we had made for his care. I was optimistic that he'd have a full recovery. The radiation completed, we could return to Pennsylvania for a month, knowing full well that we would need to be back at the VTH after that to start his chemotherapy.

I was eager to return to Pennsylvania. I felt the change of scenery would do us all good.

9
A Twist of Fate

I was right; the time in Pennsylvania had been good for all of us. I felt like I was mentally strong again—that I'd healed from the emotional drain caused by the weeks of radiation. It was good to have had the time back home, getting recharged to face the days ahead. I had been careful to ensure that Cliff didn't overdo it while recovering from the radiation. We had still taken short hikes together, enjoying the sunshine and the cool weather. Cliff was clearly back to his old self. The dermatitis at the radiation site had healed well, and a scab had formed. I'd continued to put aloe on it, and just recently, I'd noticed that the hair was starting to grow back.

While in Pennsylvania, Dick and I had gone out to dinner, and talked about our first close brush with cancer. Dick's father, Fritz, had passed away at the age of seventy-four after a brief, painful struggle with bone cancer. It had come on quickly, taking him away from us in only three short months. I remembered how hard it had been on Dick, losing Fritz so quickly after he was diagnosed, and how difficult it had been to watch him shrink away to nothing, week by week. Before cancer, Fritz had been a man of imposing stature, over six feet tall and of a very large build. I recalled the first time I'd met Fritz, and how it felt to shake his hand, which was almost three times the size of mine. Cancer had taken Fritz from us too soon, and we keenly felt the absence of this man who'd been such a presence in our lives.

Now, I was facing cancer again, this time with Cliff. I found that my memory of Fritz's battle was very much alive, and this new experience was forcing me to take a closer look at death. I pondered over it, wondering which would be the better way to die: quickly and without warning, say, from a heart attack? Or, after a long, drawn-out illness like cancer? Heart attacks do not allow you to say good-bye, but a quick death eliminates the suffering of a long illness. Cancer allows you to say your final farewells, but also makes the last months painful for everyone involved.

Ultimately, I decided there is no ideal way to die, and felt relieved that I wouldn't have to choose my fate. All I could hope for was to make the most of the days I had left on this earth—and to do my utmost to ensure the same for Cliff.

We flew back to Colorado on a chilly November day. Cliff was scheduled to start chemotherapy the next morning, but I'd come to think that perhaps it could be delayed. I'd called Dr. Selting and left her a message, and was waiting for her return call. I was sure that she'd left a message on my cell phone, or at the house.

I knew we would be landing in Lincoln, Nebraska, to refuel, and I planned to call and check my messages then. I looked down at Cliff, lying on a blanket on the floor next to me. He had started to limp just two days earlier, and I thought that maybe he'd sprained his foot or leg while running in the wet grass. I wasn't sure if he'd be getting off the plane with Jokonita and me in Lincoln, as was our custom. I had always walked Cliff and Nita during our stops in Lincoln, but that was when Cliff could still climb the stairs by himself, something he was unable to do on this trip.

Up until Cliff had started limping, he'd been doing well, showing no outward signs of pain. I had decided to wait and see if the limping got better, but after one day it had not improved. I was concerned because it was the same leg that had been treated with radiation. I'd called my vet in Pennsylvania the day before—a Sunday—and listened to a recording that indicated Dr. Karen Jones, the on-call vet, would be paged in the event of any emergencies. Usually I saw Dr. Friedlander, but I knew

Dr. Jones, and felt comfortable seeing her. I just wanted someone to look at Cliff's leg. I left a message, and a short time later got a call back telling me to bring Cliff in at 11:30.

When the call came, I was on my way out the door to meet my friend Kate for a mountain bike ride. Dick told me I should go ahead and take my ride; he would take Cliff in to see the vet. By the time I got to the place where I was to meet Kate, I knew I couldn't go for a bike ride. I had to be with Cliff. I was fighting back the tears as I explained to Kate about Cliff's limp. Kate understood and gave me a hug. I got back into the Suburban and drove as fast as I could to the vet's office, where Dr. Jones was just finishing up with another dog.

I took a seat in the waiting area next to Dick and Cliff; they had arrived just a short time before. Soon, we were called into an exam room, where Dr. Jones examined Cliff's leg and looked at the radiation site.

"I don't see any indication that Cliff has fractured a bone," the vet said. "And since he's still putting weight on it, I think that perhaps it's just sprained."

"We're leaving for Colorado tomorrow," I told her, "and I have an appointment for him at CSU, to start his chemotherapy the day after." After more discussion, we decided I should have them check Cliff's leg when we got to the VTH.

"Since I first noticed his limp, I began to give him morphine again, just once a day," I said.

"Increase it to two times a day," Dr. Jones instructed. "I want to be sure that we're keeping him as comfortable and pain-free as possible."

I nodded, and thanked her for her help as we left the exam room. I felt somewhat reassured, knowing that Dr. Jones thought it was sufficient to have the VTH staff take a look at Cliff's leg when we got to Colorado. We went ahead with our plans to fly out on Monday.

On Monday morning, Cliff had refused to put any weight on his leg, so I held him around the chest and Dick lifted his back end while we carefully carried him up the four stairs into the plane. Earlier that day while en route to the airport, Dick and I had talked about Cliff. Although we never discussed the option of "putting him down," I think Dick *wanted* to talk about it. However, this was not a conversation I was ready to have. What I wanted for Cliff was for him to be happy, pain-free, and to have the ability to run and play as he had in the past. I was still very hopeful that this injury was nothing serious, and one from which he could fully recover.

Once in Lincoln, Dick and I decided to carry Cliff off and on the plane so we could all get some fresh air. I checked my messages, and sure enough, there was one from Dr. Selting. She told me that she had set up an appointment for Cliff to be seen by Orthopedics the next morning. I was glad to hear this, and hoped that by tomorrow at this time, we would know what was wrong with Cliff's leg.

When we landed in Eagle, we again carried Cliff off the plane, and put him in the back of the Suburban. I knew that the next twenty-four hours would be a challenge for us, because our Colorado home has many stairs. Steps were everywhere—two up to the kitchen, five down to our bedroom—and that was only on the main floor. When we arrived, Dick carried Cliff up to the main level, where we stayed for most of the night, Cliff resting on the living room couch, next to me. When it was time to go to bed, I had Dick carry Cliff into the bedroom to keep him from trying to hop down the steps on three legs and possibly falling.

The next morning, we left early for our drive to Fort Collins. Dick came along this time, and when we got to the veterinary hospital, he again carried Cliff into the waiting room. During the drive to the VTH I'd received a call from Dr. Selting, telling me that orthopedic surgeon Dr. Elizabeth Pluhar would be seeing Cliff.

After we'd checked in at the front desk, we met with Dr. Pluhar right away. She calmly sat down next to us, and greeted us with a warm, friendly smile. I explained that Cliff had been doing great, but had developed the limp two days earlier. I started to tell her about our past visits to the VTH, and about Cliff's cancer, but she stopped me, saying that Dr. Selting had already briefed her on our case.

"I'd like to do some X-rays of his leg, so we can get a clear picture of what we're dealing with," Dr. Pluhar said. "I've already got him scheduled to be seen by Radiology, and they'll be coming for him shortly."

Dick and I nodded our assent, and while we were waiting, Dr. Selting came by. I was relieved to see her, and anxious to fill her in on Cliff's situation.

"Have you spoken with Dr. Pluhar yet?" she asked.

"Yes—we're just waiting for Radiology to come and get Cliff," I replied.

"After the X-rays come back, and we know what we're dealing with, we can discuss what we're going to do about the chemotherapy," Dr. Selting said.

A Radiology staff member came to take Cliff for his X-rays, and not long afterward, Dr. Pluhar brought him back out. He was hopping more than walking, using only three legs, and not putting any weight on the sore leg. Dr. Selting had joined us for the consultation. Dr. Pluhar explained that on the X-ray, it looked like Cliff had a problem with some of the bones in his knee, and possibly, also a ruptured cruciate ligament.

"The bones that work together and hinge in the knee are slipping," she said, "and that's probably what is causing the pain. Instead of just repairing the cruciate ligament," she continued, "surgeons can reshape the bone to make it fit better with the other bones. The procedure is called a tibial plateau leveling osteotomy, or TPLO," Dr. Pluhar said.

"That sounds complicated," I said, and expressed my hesitation about having it done.

"It's been successfully performed many times," Dr. Pluhar assured us.

Upon further explanation, I learned that the surgery involves making a cut in the tibia (the shin bone), and repositioning the top of the bone so that it is at a different angle, more level than it was before. After the procedure, the forces on the knee joint are more balanced while bearing weight, meaning that the knee no longer needs the support of the ruptured ligament to keep it in line. This procedure is patented and can only be performed by certified surgeons.

I glanced over at Dick, who gave me a look that clearly said, "It's your call." Considering that this was probably the best possible fix for Cliff's leg, we agreed to have the surgery done. I wanted to schedule it right away, but because it was close to the Thanksgiving holiday, we would have to wait a week. I wasn't happy about this, but realized that as long as Cliff was not in any pain, we could manage.

After Dr. Pluhar left, Dr. Selting talked to us about the next step in Cliff's treatment schedule. "Chemo will have to wait until after Cliff has recovered from the surgery," she said. "For now, keep Cliff on the morphine, and also, start him on carprofen to help with the pain. Keep in touch with me over the next week, to let me know how Cliff's doing," she added.

"I will—and I'll see you next week when we return for the surgery," I said.

When we got home, I started thinking about how I could make the house more accessible to Cliff. He was slipping and falling on the hardwood floors, and continued to have great difficulty climbing the stairs. He didn't seem to have a problem on the carpets, however, so I decided to create a path through the house for him to walk on. I found some rubber carpet mats in the storage room and cut them into pieces to place between the area rugs. To keep them in position, I used red mechanical tape to secure them to the hardwood floor. Once I'd completed a small pathway, I called Cliff over to see if he would walk on it. He seemed apprehensive at first, especially on the two steps up to the kitchen, but he tried it. He was still hobbling on three legs, but at least now he wasn't slipping and falling. Before I knew it, I had created a maze of very pretty Oriental rugs connected to each other with rubber mats that ran throughout the house. It looked rather strange, but I didn't care; it would be functional.

Amy, Andy, and Chase, now seven months old, were due to arrive the next day to celebrate Thanksgiving with us. Because Dick would be leaving for Pennsylvania on business, Amy and Chase would accompany me to Fort Collins the following week. I was getting anxious about the surgery, but I was ready to get back to the VTH. I knew the sooner they fixed his leg, the better off Cliff would be. We would be dealing with the surgery first, but the question of when he would start the chemo remained unanswered. I was glad that Amy and Chase would be going with me this time. I knew that having them there would make it easier—at the very least, they would help to occupy my time, taking my mind off my worries.

On the Monday morning following Thanksgiving, Dick and Andy left, and I spent the day getting organized for our trip to Fort Collins. I had no idea how long I was going to be there this time, but I was prepared to stay as long as I needed to. I packed the Suburban with Chase's ExerSaucer and portable playpen, and of course, my road bike, which always goes with me. I used bungee cords to secure everything to one side of the cargo area, so as to leave plenty of room for Cliff and Jokonita. Normally, they had the entire cargo area, but this time, a third of it was taken up with other items.

We'd be staying at the Marriott Residence Inn again this time, as it was very functional for us. Our suite included a small kitchen, where I could prepare meals for Cliff and Jokonita. I was well aware that when we started the chemo, Cliff could lose his appetite. I knew that I might have to entice him to eat with the special dinners I'd make for him. I also liked staying there because of the warm welcome I received from the staff; it was a homey environment, and eased some of the tension I felt from being in a strange town.

Before staying at the Marriott, I hadn't known a soul in Fort Collins—except for the people I'd met at the VTH—and it was nice to see the same friendly faces each time I checked in. There was a social area off the lobby where people mingled, and the staff served appetizers and beverages there at night. It was also where everyone gathered for breakfast. It was nice to get out of my room and be around others. Plus, in the evenings I could take Cliff and Jokonita down with me if Cliff was feeling well enough.

During one stay there, I'd met and become friends with two women who also had dogs that had cancer and were being treated at CSU. Carla, from Aspen, Colorado, had a white, long-haired standard poodle named Cassidy, who had cancer in her foot. Jackie, from California, had a black puli named Dooley, who had cancer in his spine. We shared the same fears and concerns, and drew strength from each other. Back at the hotel at night, we would often cook dinner together for our "fur babies." The evenings were often the hardest, and we agreed it was nice to be able to relax over a glass of wine and talk with someone who understood what you were going through. We were all grateful to be together and have the chance to support each other. During my early days at the VTH, I had found it difficult to talk to others in the waiting room. Unable to actually voice my fears and concerns, I was probably still very much in denial about what was happening to Cliff. These evenings with Carla and Jackie helped me to realize the importance of sharing this experience with others who were going through the same steps, and feeling the same emotions.

When I got to the VTH the morning after our return to Fort Collins, I was told that the surgery would take a few hours, and that they'd call me on my cell phone when Cliff was in recovery. Before I turned Cliff over to them, I leaned down and gave him a hug. "They're going to fix your leg, and in no time, you'll be playing with Jokonita again," I said.

I smiled at the thought, and gave him one more hug and a kiss on the top of his head. I watched as he hobbled down the hall, hoping that this would all be over soon.

I had left Jokonita at the hotel with Amy and Chase, so I headed back to get them for a few hours of shopping. When I got to the hotel, Amy and Chase were dressed and ready to go. I took Jokonita for a short walk, and then we all climbed into the Suburban and went to Old Town. It was a beautiful, sunny fall day, and after a few hours of shopping, we decided to eat lunch in a restaurant with an outside patio. I kept my phone on the table, very anxious for it to ring, which it did soon after we'd finished lunch.

It was Dr. Pluhar, and the news was not good.

"Cliff was prepped and ready for surgery, and we had just taken another X-ray of his leg," she said. "What we saw this time was not what we saw only eight days ago." Her tone was ominous. "I think Cliff has cancer in the bone in his knee, and this is what has been causing the pain," Dr. Pluhar said. "I don't think there is a tear to the cruciate ligament, so I've canceled the surgery."

I stood there, speechless, as my phone beeped in with another call. I quickly switched over and found myself talking to Dr. Selting. Her voice revealed how disturbed she was by Dr. Pluhar's news. She asked me to come back quickly so we could discuss our options.

Amy, Chase, and I headed back to the car. The tears in my eyes made it nearly impossible for me to drive. I couldn't believe this was happening. *Bone cancer—the same disease that had taken Fritz from us. Is that what they are telling me Cliff has?*

When I got back, Dr. Selting took me into the exam room and showed me the two sets of X-rays—the set taken today, and the set taken eight days ago. The difference in the X-rays was very obvious. There now was an area on the bone that looked like it was moth-eaten, plain and simple.

"Taking a second X-ray was just normal procedure for the type of surgery we'd planned," Dr. Selting said. "It enables us to take some measurements and calculate angles in order to correct the bone. If we'd planned to do a different type of surgery," she added, "we wouldn't have taken the second X-ray, and then, we wouldn't have known about the cancer until it was too late." (Both Dr. Pluhar and Dr. Selting later commented on the good fortune of this remarkable chain of events. If the surgery had not been delayed because of the Thanksgiving holiday, it would have been done right after the initial consultation with Dr. Pluhar. Considering the ultimate diagnosis, this would have been an extraneous procedure.)

The most disturbing part of the news was that Cliff's original cancer was anal sac adenocarcinoma, and it was unlikely that it had spread to the bone. It was more likely that this was a *second* type of cancer.

"We're doing a biopsy on a piece of the bone, and it's being rushed to the lab," Dr. Selting said. "We're waiting for the results now." I stood there in stunned silence, trying to comprehend what she was telling me. Giving me an understanding glance, she left for a moment to find Cliff, bringing him back to me a few minutes later.

"I'm going to see if the biopsy is back yet," she said.

I nodded, sitting there numbly, hugging Cliff. *I'm not going to let them amputate your leg,* I thought. I'd seen many dogs running around the VTH with only three legs, and although they probably did just fine, I was not going to do that to Cliff. There had to be something else we could do.

Soon Dr. Selting came back in the exam room. I could tell by her face that the news was bad. "The biopsy confirmed that it is indeed a second type of cancer, a bone cancer called osteosarcoma," she said. "The lesion we saw in the knee is at the distal femur—the end of the thigh bone—and it's caused the collapse of the condyle, the rounded part at the end of the bone. This makes it a pathologic fracture," Dr. Selting said, "one where the bone has broken down and collapsed because of the cancer inside it."

I listened as she told me the details. When she mentioned the possibility of amputating his leg, I immediately said no—Dick and I had decided in the very beginning that we were only going to continue on a path that would *improve* Cliff's quality of life, and amputation would not do that.

She then told me about a procedure that spared the limb, called a "flip 'n' nuc" (pronounced *nuke*), or an intraoperative radiation spare (IOR). This type of surgery had been performed in the past, with good results. With this procedure, the cancerous bone is cut away from the surrounding healthy muscle and soft tissue. The part of the bone with the cancer is gently rotated out of the body so that the cancerous area is pulled away from the normal tissues, while leaving the joint intact. The area with the cancer then receives a very high dose of radiation; this is possible because they do not have to worry about damaging the surrounding normal tissues, since they have been moved out of the path of the radiation. This is all done under anesthesia in sterile operating conditions. The bone is then rotated back into the body to its original position and a bone plate is used to repair the cut in the bone. The soft tissues are brought back to their original positions, and everything is sutured together.

"There are two surgeons at the VTH who have done this procedure," Dr. Selting continued. We continued to discuss this option, and decided that if possible, these doctors should work together as a team to perform the surgery on Cliff. Dr. Selting said, "Before the surgery is done, it would be prudent to do a bone scan to be sure this is an isolated lesion, and that there are no others on Cliff's skeletal system."

"I feel certain this is an isolated case," I said. "But . . . all right—let's go ahead and do the bone scan."

The scan was scheduled for the next day. This procedure required that Cliff be injected with a nuclear substance, which takes twenty-four hours to be eliminated from his body. Because of the substance's radioactivity, Cliff would have to spend the night at the VTH, and I would not be able to see him until he had been "cleared" of the substance. I was very upset at the thought of leaving him for twenty-four hours, but I knew I had no choice.

"You can go ahead and take Cliff back to the hotel with you now," Dr. Selting said gently. "Just bring him back early tomorrow morning." I nodded, a quiet "Thank you" all I could manage. I was not sure what to think; I only knew we were facing more questions than answers.

Amy and Chase were in the waiting room. I quickly explained to Amy what I'd just been told as we headed back to the hotel so Cliff could get some rest. I was sure that just being in the VTH was exhausting for him. I wanted him to be well rested for the bone scan the next day.

I was back at the VTH early the next morning, prepared to leave Cliff in Dr. Selting's care.

"It will be much later in the day before I have the results of the bone scan," she said. "I'll call your cell phone the minute they're in."

As usual, I hugged Cliff and told him that it was going to be okay. Knowing that I would not be able to see him for twenty-four long hours, I explained that he would have to spend the night there. "I'll be back to get you first thing in the morning," I said, trying to inject a cheerful tone into my voice.

Dr. Selting—Kim, as we were now on a first-name basis—assured me they would take great care of Cliff, and she'd call me later in the day.

"We're going to Estes Park for the day," I said. "I think a change of scenery will do us all good. I'm not sure how well my cell phone will work there, but if I don't hear from you by three o'clock, I'll call the VTH from a land phone."

She nodded. I knew she understood how I felt; we'd come to know each other well in a relatively short time. Going through something like this together tends to bring people closer. I bade farewell to Cliff, and made my way out the door. I was surprised at how composed I was.

Amy, Chase, and Nita were already in the Suburban, waiting for me, so we headed to Estes Park. I had never been there before, and was looking forward to spending some time with Amy and Chase. In a little over an hour we were walking through the shops and galleries. At one point, I heard a commotion on the street; walking outside to investigate, I saw a herd of elk on the hillside above us. I wondered if that was a regular occurrence, and found that I enjoyed the distraction.

We took Chase to a photo studio that specialized in creating old-time photographs. He looked so cute sitting in an old tin washtub wearing only his diaper, a cowboy hat, and a scarf around his neck. After the photo session, we took a break for lunch. All the while, I kept checking my phone. Even though I had a full signal, I had yet to hear from Kim.

At three o'clock, I decided to call Kim to see how things were going. I wondered if maybe the bone scan had been delayed. I knew that emergencies often popped up at the VTH, causing the schedule to shift. I had the number programmed into my phone, so in a matter of seconds I was connected. When Kim answered, I immediately sensed that something was very wrong.

"I've been trying to get up the nerve to call you," she said. "I'm afraid the news isn't good."

My heart started pounding.

"I'm so sorry, JoAnne," Kim said. "The bone scan shows many lesions on Cliff's skeletal system."

"I'll be there as quickly as I can," I said, and hung up.

Amy knew it was serious just by the tremor in my voice. I told her briefly what Kim had said. I was unable to say much; my throat was dry, and I was finding it hard to speak. We gathered up Chase and our packages and walked quickly to the car.

The drive back felt unreal. I kept thinking to myself, *How bad can this be? Why can't we just radiate them all?* I'm not sure if I was in some sort of denial, or in shock. My mind was whirling as I tried to grasp what Kim had said. I'm afraid that most of the ride passed in a blur.

When I got to the VTH, Kim was waiting for me. She took me into one of the exam rooms, where the scan was already hanging on the wall. It looked like an X-ray, except that the lesions showed up as bright spots because of the radioactive substance that had been injected into Cliff.

"These are the lesions I was talking about," Kim said, looking troubled as she watched for my reaction.

I can't believe this, I thought, even though it was laid out right there for me to see. I didn't know what to say to Kim. I looked at Amy and Chase, who had followed me into the room. I felt bad that Amy had to witness this; she had tears in her eyes. Up until this point, I'd been able to keep a lot of things to myself—especially my deepest fears. I hadn't wanted to worry my family. But there was no denying now that this was very bad news indeed. I found words hard to come by, and stood there for a moment in silence. I looked at Chase, and felt thankful that he was there with us. He would be the little angel who would help us through the difficult evening ahead.

I turned back to Kim, and steeled myself to ask some of the tough questions.

"Can't we radiate all of the lesions?" I asked.

"No," she said sadly. "His body can't take that much radiation. There are lesions on his spine, his front shoulder, his ribs and back leg—even on his tail. It appears that the cancer has spread throughout his whole skeletal system," she said. "The only good news is that none of his organs have been affected. His lungs and his lymph nodes are still all clear."

"I'm not giving up," I told Kim firmly. "There has to be something else that we can do. I'm open to *anything* that will save Cliff's life. There are no options I won't explore."

I think Kim was at a loss for words. I felt she wanted to give me at least a shred of good news, or at the very least, some hope, but nothing came.

"I'm sorry the news is so bad," Kim said.

I wondered then about what she really thought. *Did she think Cliff was going to die?* I never asked. A part of me still felt that Cliff was going to be okay. Kim reached out to hug me, and I felt the tears start to well up in my eyes. I knew that I had to get out of there. I was not ready to have this conversation with her. I didn't want to know what she thought about Cliff's time frame. I was not ready to stop trying.

I turned to Amy and said, "Let's go." I told Kim that I would be back first thing in the morning, and added on our way out, my voice catching on the words, "Please find something that can help Cliff."

I left a part of me at the VTH that night. Amy, Chase, Jokonita, and I went back to the hotel. All evening I found the need to take Jokonita out for walks. I needed to be outside, needed the natural world. I watched the sun fade over the mountain, and then later, saw the stars appear in the sky. I was very calm and determined. I was sure that there had to be another choice. I asked for help—prayed for a miracle.

The next morning I got up with a reaffirmed attitude. I was determined that I was not going to let cancer win—not without a fight. Up until the day before, I'd had no idea how bad it was, but now, I had a clear picture. Cliff could only survive this if I stayed strong and stood firmly by his side.

When I got to the VTH, Kim told me that Cliff had been cleared of the nuclear substance used in his bone scan, and he was waiting for me in an exam room. I could tell she wanted to talk to me, so I followed her down the hallway, toward the room where Cliff was waiting. I glanced in the exam room window before we went in. Cliff looked amazing; he was lying there calmly, waiting for me. When I opened the door, he came running to me, jumping and yelping as if he were still a puppy. The love we shared filled the room, and I was overjoyed. Kim smiled. I could tell she felt it too.

I turned to Kim, my resolve strengthened. "I want to explore any and every option we have, Kim."

At first she did not say much—just looked at me, her eyes kind. "I'll see what I can find," she said finally. I sensed that she may have already been looking into some options, but nothing she was ready to share with me yet.

After Cliff and I had enjoyed our reunion, I took him outside to see Amy, Chase, and Jokonita. Everyone had been missing him, and I knew that Nita did not understand why he hadn't been at the hotel with us last night. I wanted her to see him, to see that he was okay. They nuzzled and licked each other, happy to be together again.

I brought Cliff back inside and took my usual seat in the waiting room. We were only there for a very short time when a young woman named Chloe came by and kneeled down to pet Cliff. I'd never met her before, but she clearly knew Cliff, and was fond of him. "I'm so sorry to hear the news," Chloe said. "I was on orthopedic rotation this week, and I just met Cliff a few days ago." She had tears in her eyes.

I smiled at her. "It's going to be okay," I said. "Cliff is going to okay. We are going to fight this disease."

She smiled back and said good-bye, wishing us luck.

I couldn't tell whether or not she believed me. I knew that one of the many hurdles we'd have to face in the weeks to come would be convincing others that Cliff could get through this.

A little while later, Kim came back to talk to me, and I could tell that something had changed. She was ready to move on to the next step in our fight to save Cliff. "As I said earlier, there are too many sites to irradiate," Kim began. "If we tried that, the radiation would kill him. I discussed this with our radiation therapist, and we've decided to radiate two areas: the one on his knee, to alleviate the pain, and a spot on his spine." She looked at me, making sure I understood. I nodded, and she went on.

"We're going to start the chemotherapy with two different types of drugs, one for each type of cancer. Both the radiation and the chemotherapy will start next week," Kim said.

She then told me about another drug called pamidronate, which had been approved by the FDA a few years earlier. "As far as I know, it's only been used with human cancer patients," Kim said, "but I think it might be worth trying on Cliff. It's in a class of drugs called bisphosphonates, and it's also referred to as a 'bone strengthener,' since it reduces the breakdown of the bones, fortifying them so the cancer cannot spread and grow."

I was very excited to hear about this drug. "I'd like to try it on Cliff," I said, feeling the first real stirrings of hope since I'd heard the results of the bone scan. This was something we could do—*right now.*

"It's very expensive," Kim said. "About five hundred dollars a dose— and we'd have to order it from a human cancer center."

"That's okay," I said. "Let's do it—as soon as possible."

Months earlier, Kim had given me an estimate of the expenses associated with treating Cliff's cancer: surgery, hospital stays, chemotherapy, radiation, and miscellaneous things like medications. At the time, I'd told her that I would do whatever it took to help Cliff, and I didn't care about the cost. I still felt the same way, but thanked her for keeping me fully informed. I felt fortunate to have the resources available to pay for Cliff's care, knowing full well that not everyone did. I had never purchased pet insurance, and was not sure what it would have covered if I had done so.

Kim added that Cliff would be the first dog at CSU to receive pamidronate. She cautioned that nothing had yet been published about its use in treating dogs, and she did not know of any other hospitals that had used this drug in treating animals.

"I don't care," I said. "I still want to try it."

Kim nodded. We would move forward with the new plan of action, which called for Cliff to get radiation on his knee and spine, four doses of each chemotherapy drug, and monthly doses of the pamidronate. I felt very comfortable with the course of treatment, and after setting up Cliff's appointments for the following week, I was feeling quite positive.

I said good-bye to Kim, and told her that I would see her next week.

She hugged me, saying, "You're the most optimistic pet owner I've ever had. I really admire your ability to put your emotions aside when you need to make decisions about Cliff's care." I smiled, and knew in my heart that there would be some good days ahead for us. I was now ready to head back to the mountains for a few days of rest. I knew it would be good for Cliff to have a break after everything he'd been through. Amy and Chase would soon be heading back to Florida, and next week when I returned, it would be just Cliff, Nita, and me.

10

Chemotherapy and Pamidronate

DECEMBER 2000

December had arrived, and I was thankful the weather was still in our favor. We hadn't had many bad storms yet, and for the most part, the roads had remained passable. I knew this could change at a moment's notice, and I was hoping that this drive to Fort Collins would be uneventful. They were calling for snow later in the day, but I was leaving early, in hopes that I'd get over Vail Pass before it arrived.

Cliff was scheduled to receive radiation on his knee and spine, and he would also be receiving one of the chemotherapy dugs, Adriamycin (also known as doxorubicin). Because the Adriamycin did not take long to administer, he could get it after his radiation treatment. I needed to have Cliff there by 10:00 A.M., and the doctors had said it would take about three hours, all told. With Cliff's inability to get around well, I'd been limiting how much time he spent outside. I was trying not to put added stress on his three usable legs. When I got to the VTH, I took Cliff inside and waited for Kim to come meet us. She joined us with her customary warm smile. "How did the weekend go?" she asked.

"It went well, thanks," I said, glad to see her. "Cliff didn't seem to get any worse; he's pretty much the same as he was last week."

Kim gave me a bit more information about Adriamycin, the chemotherapy drug Cliff would be getting today. "Chemotherapy in animals is generally different from that of human cancer patients," she said, "since animal patients have fewer side effects than humans. Adriamycin is a full-spectrum chemotherapy drug that's been used for decades to fight many forms of cancer. It's a slow intravenous drip directly into the vein, and takes approximately twenty minutes to administer. There are some possible side

75

effects," Kim cautioned, "the most common of which are the reduction of white blood cells, and stomach or intestinal discomfort.

"Before each dose, Cliff will receive a CBC to make sure his white blood count is at the appropriate level. Again, I want to reassure you that most animal patients do not exhibit many side effects from the chemo. Cliff will be ready in about three hours, and you can either call me, or just stop back in," she concluded.

"Okay, I'll probably just come back later," I said, leaning down to give Cliff a big hug and kiss. I felt very comfortable with all the information Kim had given me, and as always, that I was leaving Cliff in good hands.

Jokonita and I spent a good part of the morning at the lake, enjoying each other's company. Although it was December, it was still quite warm in Fort Collins. With daily highs still in the fifties and sixties, it was quite pleasant.

I wasn't anticipating that anything would go wrong at the VTH, and headed back there at 1:00 P.M. To my delight, Kim told me that Cliff had just finished the chemo, and was ready to go home. His CBC was fine, and the radiation had also gone well. Kim asked me to be there at 9:00 the next morning so they could start the other chemo drug. She told me that the Cisplatin would take much longer to administer, and Cliff would need to be there all day. Because he would be confined for such a long time the next day, I loaded Cliff in the Suburban and we went back to the lake so he could have some time in the sunshine and fresh air.

The next morning when I got to the VTH, Kim met us once again in the waiting area. She talked about the chemo drug that Cliff would be getting that day, explaining that the worst potential side effect of Cisplatin was kidney damage.

"To minimize this risk, Cliff will receive intravenous fluids for four hours prior to receiving the Cisplatin, and then again afterwards for an hour, to flush his kidneys," Kim said. "Then, another CBC will be done, as well as a blood urea nitrogen—called a BUN—to check his kidney functions. It will be around seven P.M. before Cliff will be ready to go home," Kim said.

As always before leaving, I gave Cliff a big hug and kiss, and told him I'd be back for him soon. It seemed that he'd grown accustomed to the VTH, and he walked away with Kim as I sat there, waiting for them to be out of sight before I left.

At 1:00 P.M., I called Kim to see how things were going. She said things were right on schedule for Cliff to be ready to go home at 7:00 P.M.

At around 5:00 P.M., I received a message from Kim telling me that there had been a complication. I could hardly imagine what could have happened. I rushed to the VTH immediately.

Once I'd arrived, Kim explained that Cliff had been resting comfortably while the chemo was being administered. "A vet student was monitoring Cliff, and periodically checking on him," Kim said. "Apparently, when the student was out of the room, Cliff started to move around and the catheter pulled loose. Instead of the chemo drug going directly into his vein, it leaked between the skin and the soft tissue in his leg."

Kim went on to explain that because of this, there was now great potential for soft tissue damage. This was particularly disturbing because the strong, healthy back leg was the one that was affected.

When I first saw Cliff, I could tell right away that his leg was very swollen with fluid, from his foot all the way up his leg. Kim was obviously upset that this had happened. Cliff's body would eventually eliminate the drug through his urine, but it might take days for this to happen, and he would have to be closely monitored throughout. Kim recommended that I stay in town during the monitoring process.

Cliff had been unhooked from the catheter, and Kim said that I could take him back to the hotel. I needed to bring him back to the VTH the next morning at 7:00 so they could check his leg.

I left thinking there had to be something else that could be done. I couldn't just sit and wait for his body to eliminate the drug. I knew I had to act fast, so I called my friend Kate back in Pennsylvania. She was into all kinds of natural remedies. I remembered that she had once accidentally slammed her hand in the door of her van. It was quite swollen, so she had made a poultice and applied it to her hand to draw out the fluids. It worked! I knew that if anyone could tell me what to do, she was the one.

Although Kate usually turned off her phone in the evenings, on this night, she happened to answer my call. I told her what had happened, and she sent me to the health food store for some castor oil and wool cloth. She told me to apply the castor oil to Cliff's leg, wrap it in the wool cloth, and then in plastic to prevent seepage. I had some plastic grocery bags that I tore open for this purpose.

After I'd gathered the necessary items, I had Cliff lie on some towels that I'd spread out on the floor. I then rubbed the castor oil into his entire leg, carefully wrapping the leg in the wool cloth and plastic to take care of the seepage, which was already starting. I was careful not to wrap it too tightly, and I secured the plastic with some vet wrap—a sticky, tapelike material that binds together like Velcro—which held everything in place. I helped Cliff get onto the bed and had him lie down on a thickly folded blanket to catch any seepage.

I sat down next to him and settled in for the next few hours, watching TV. Jokonita wanted to be close to us, so she hopped up onto the bed, too. I could tell she sensed that something was wrong with Cliff. We stayed in the room all night, with minimal activity.

When I got up at 6:00 the next morning, I saw nothing short of a miracle. I carefully removed the vet wrap, the plastic, and the soaked wool cloth that had been on Cliff's leg for almost twelve hours. The castor oil

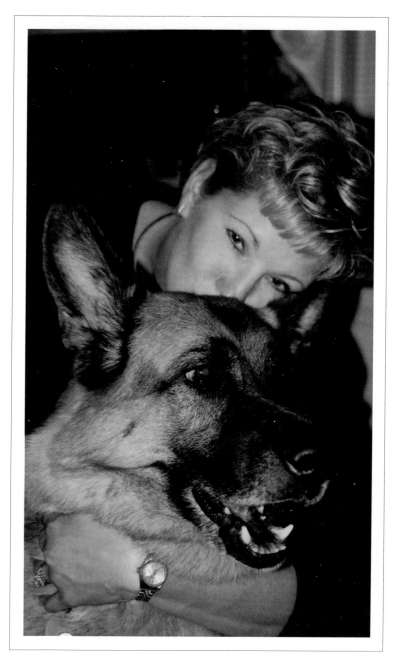

JoAnne & Cliff

MY FAVORITE PICTURE OF US
PHOTO BY GINA HARRISON (GOOD FRIEND)
1997

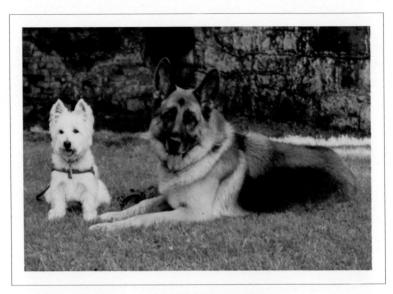

Kenzie & Cliff

PHOTO BY LETTIE DAVIS (DICK'S AUNT)
PENNSYLVANIA 1997

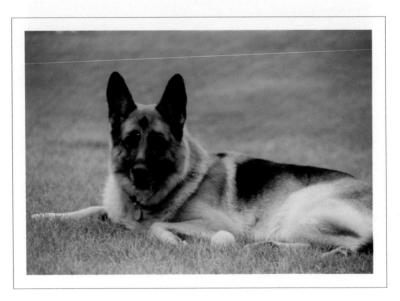

Cliff with Tennis Ball

PHOTO BY LETTIE DAVIS (DICK'S AUNT)
PENNSYLVANIA 1997

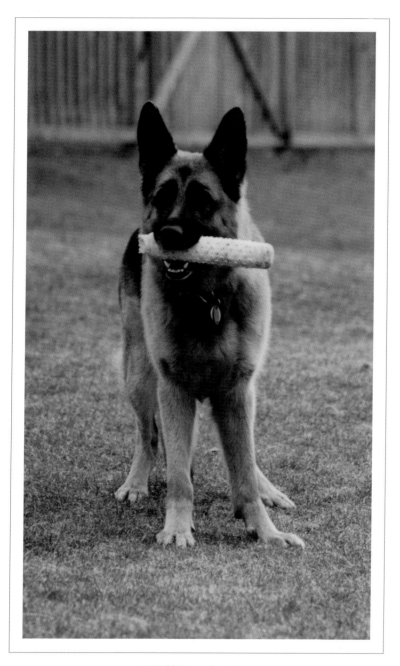

Cliff Retrieving

PENNSYLVANIA 1997

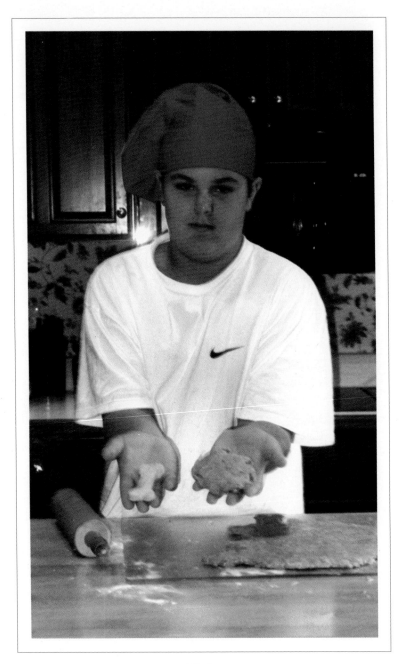

Blake

BAKING BISCUITS FOR CLIFF
PENNSYLVANIA 1997

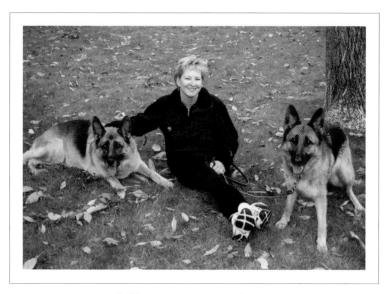

Cliff, JoAnne & Jokonita

THE DAY JOKONITA JOINED OUR FAMILY
PENNSYLVANIA, OCTOBER 1999

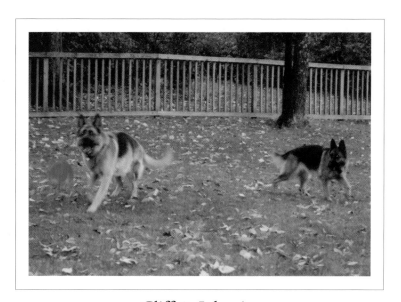

Cliff & Jokonita

THEIR FIRST DAY PLAYING TOGETHER
PENNSYLVANIA, OCTOBER 1999

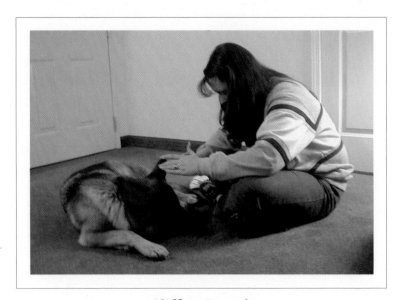

Cliff & Brenda

PERFORMING REIKI
FORT COLLINS, COLORADO 2000

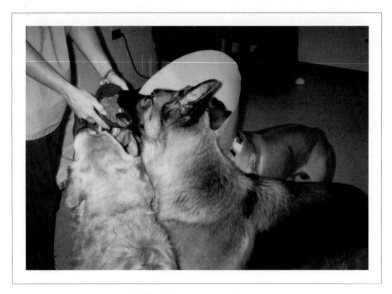

Cliff Sharing a Snack

WITH OTHER PATIENTS
CSU VTH 2000

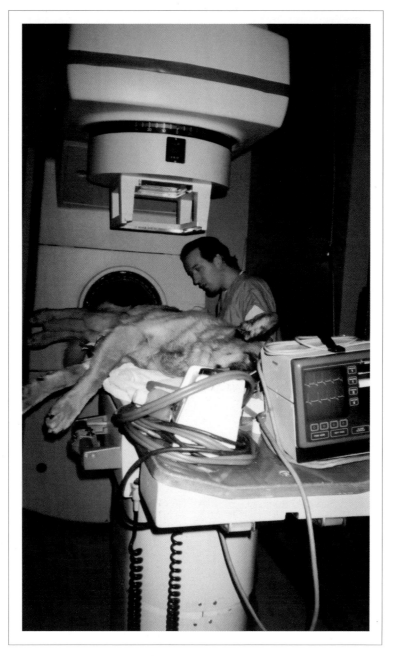

Cliff Getting Radiation

SEDATED DURING TREATMENT
CSU VTH 2000

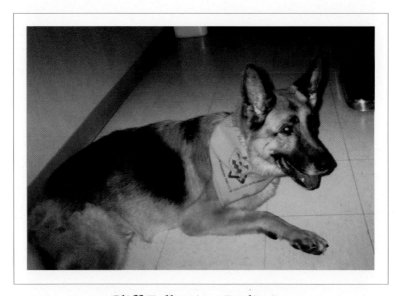

Cliff Following Radiation

JUST AFTER HIS LAST RADIATION TREATMENT
CSU VTH 2000

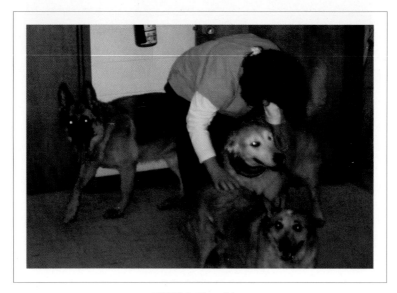

Cliff Mingling

WITH OTHER PATIENTS
CSU VTH 2000

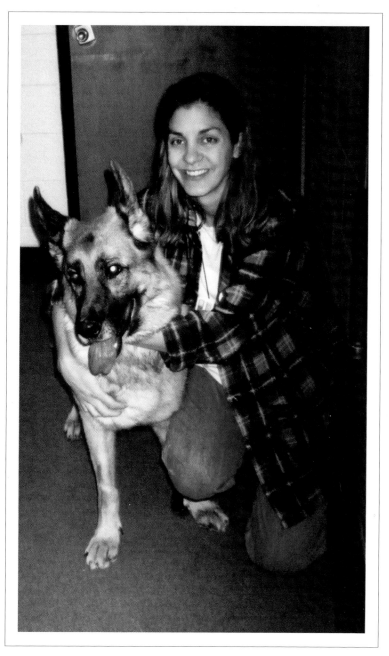

Cliff & Dr. Kim Selting

CSU VTH 2000

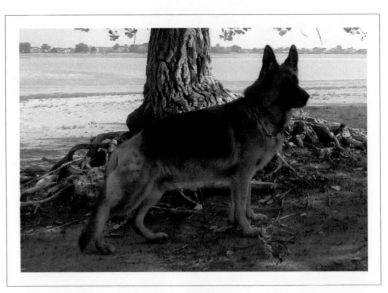

Cliff

SHAVED BACK END WITH RADIATION X'S
BOYD LAKE 2000

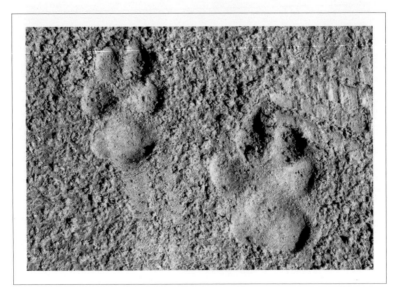

Cliff's Paw Prints

BOYD LAKE 2000

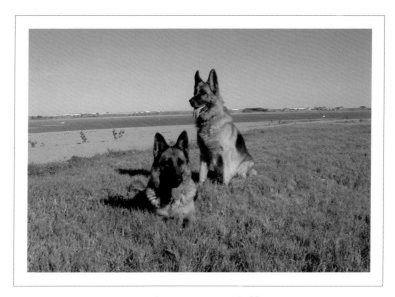

Jokonita & Cliff

RELAXING BY THE WATER
BOYD LAKE 2000

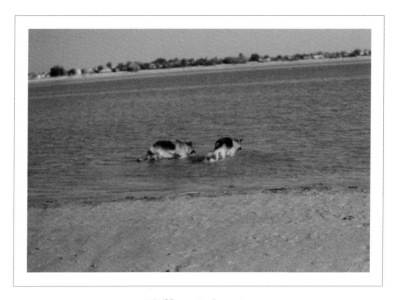

Cliff & Jokonita

PLAYING IN THE WATER
BOYD LAKE 2000

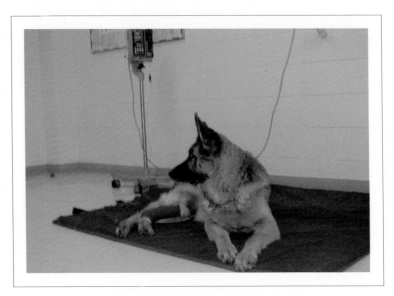

Cliff During Chemotherapy
A PAINLESS PROCEDURE
CSU VTH 2000

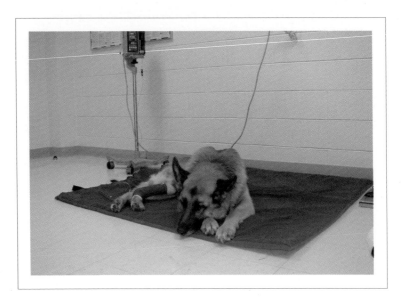

Cliff During Chemotherapy
RESTING AND CALM
CSU VTH 2000

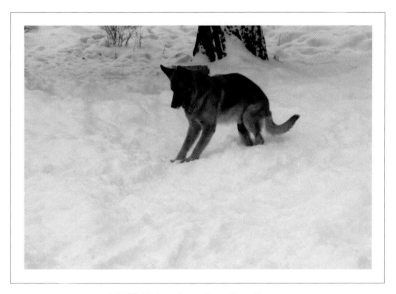

Cliff Digging in the Snow

BACK RIGHT LEG SHAVED
STILL PLAYFUL AFTER SURGERY
COLORADO 2000

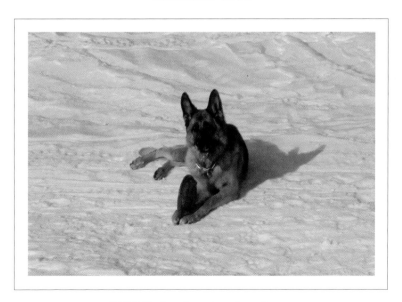

Cliff Relaxing in the Snow

SHAVED BACK LEG AND KNEE
COLORADO 2000

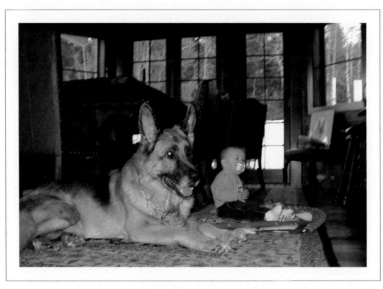

Cliff & Chase

BACK LEG SHAVED
VERY FRIENDLY WITH CHILDREN
COLORADO 2000

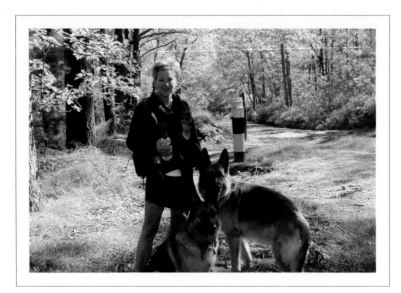

JoAnne, Cliff (right) & Jokonita Hiking

PENNSYLVANIA
FALL 2000

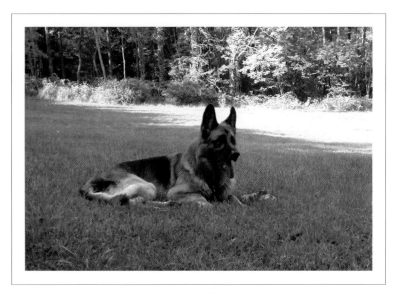

Cliff
ONE YEAR AFTER SURGERY
HAIR GROWN BACK, SLIGHT CHANGE IN TAIL
PENNSYLVANIA, FALL 2001

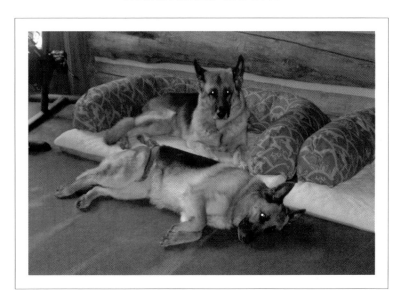

Cliff & Jokonita in Bed
JOKONITA WEARING PANTS (IN HEAT)
COLORADO 2001

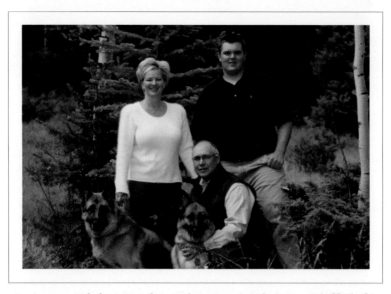

JoAnne, Blake, Dick, Jokonita (right) & Cliff (left)
PHOTO BY TOM MCCARTHY (VAIL VALLEY PORTRAITS)
COLORADO, JULY 2001

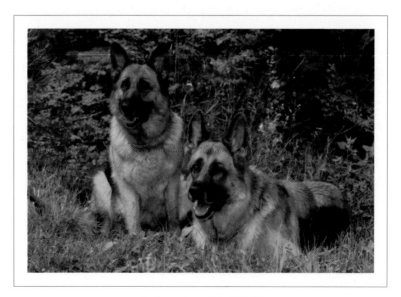

Jokonita & Cliff
GRAY HAIR ON BACK AFTER RADIATION TO SPINE
PHOTO BY TOM MCCARTHY (VAIL VALLEY PORTRAITS)
COLORADO, JULY 2001

had actually drawn the fluid out of his leg. I estimated that the swelling was down by 95 percent.

I quickly loaded Cliff and Jokonita into the Suburban and drove to the VTH. Kim was amazed when she saw Cliff, and listened closely as I told her what I had done. She called for Dr. Withrow. I had a feeling she'd talked with him about what had happened the day before, and she wanted him to see the improvement. From the expression on his face, I could tell he was very surprised to see that the swelling was nearly gone. I explained my home remedy, and with a slightly stunned expression, he said, "Whatever works."

"We'll still want to check Cliff again tomorrow," Kim said. "But from what I'm seeing today, it's likely he'll be able to leave town then." I was delighted.

Sure enough, when Kim saw Cliff the next day, she said that after he'd received the bone-strengthening pamidronate, he could return to the mountains with me. We were all hopeful that this drug would work as well for him as it had been working in human cancer patients. I was, however, concerned about another accident happening with the catheter.

"Would it be possible for me to sit with Cliff while he is receiving his treatments from now on?" I asked Kim.

"That would be fine," Kim replied.

So, I sat on the mat next to Cliff on the tiny exam-room floor. I watched the bag that was attached to the pump, which was attached to him, and thought about the drug in the bag. *How I wish it had been available when Fritz had bone cancer!* That was only five years before, and although no cure had been found for cancer, at least they were constantly finding new treatments that helped—small steps to improve the quality of life.

I was happy that Cliff would be the first dog to use this drug at the VTH. I hoped it would work, and that others would be helped by what we were learning. I was glad that my persistence had led Kim to find this drug. Kim and I made a good team, although at times I'm sure she wondered where I found my unlimited supply of optimism. I knew she was a good doctor, and I had total faith in her and the team of experts she worked with in this hospital. We were all in this together. I felt I would trust them with my life—just as I was trusting them at this moment with Cliff's.

Cliff continued to rest calmly next to me, lying on his side while the drug was being administered. I was thankful that I could be there to comfort him. I glanced down and smiled at him, occasionally reaching over to stroke his forehead. I knew that with me there, he would rest comfortably throughout the entire treatment. Just around the time when the last few drops were flowing into the tube, Kim came back in.

"How's my patient doing?" she asked.

"Just fine," I said.

As she unhooked the catheter from Cliff, she asked me to keep an eye on his leg over the weekend, and to be on the lookout for any soft tissue damage. I told her that I would, smiling to myself; I knew in my heart that the worst was over. By stepping outside of the box, outside of mainline medical procedures, I had prevented a potentially damaging situation. I was pleased, and also now on a mission to look at other alternative treatments that could possibly help Cliff.

Kim bent down to hug Cliff, and then she hugged me. I smiled, and told her that we'd be back next week.

11
Acupuncture and Reiki

DECEMBER 2000

When we next returned to the VTH, I had scheduled Cliff for acupuncture, in addition to the radiation, chemo, and pamidronate. Kim had given me the name of Dr. Narda Robinson, an acupuncturist at the VTH. After we'd finished Cliff's chemotherapy, we would meet with her for the first time. I was very excited about trying acupuncture, and hopeful that it would help Cliff just as it had helped me when I had tendinitis in my elbow. Dick had also been cured of migraines with the help of acupuncture treatments.

On our first day back, Cliff was resting comfortably in the exam room, so I asked the receptionist if it would be all right for Dr. Robinson to meet with us there. She said that would be fine. When Dr. Robinson joined us, I stood up and shook her hand, introducing myself and Cliff. She sat down on the floor next to Cliff, reached in the pocket of her white lab coat, and pulled out a dog biscuit. She asked me if Cliff could have it, and when I said yes, she gave it to him. He ate it with gusto, and then sniffed her pocket, looking for more.

I began to fill Dr. Robinson in on the events of recent months, including what had happened the past week with the chemo drug leaking into the soft tissue of Cliff's leg. I told her how I'd used a castor-oil wrap to draw out the fluid, and explained that I was interested in trying anything that might help Cliff.

Dr. Robinson started by telling me that acupuncture was used to help with the side effects of cancer treatments. "It can help to strengthen Cliff's immune system," she said, "and may also help with nausea." As she reached into her bag to pull out a box of needles, she looked at me.

"How do you think Cliff will handle this?" she asked.

"He'll be fine," I said. "As long as I'm next to him, I think he'll just lie here calmly while you work on him." I knew that my presence would reassure Cliff.

As Dr. Robinson started to put the needles in, I gently rubbed Cliff's head, telling him that everything was fine, that she was there to help him. While she worked on Cliff, I told her about some of the things I'd started to give him, one being a supplement called IP-6 and Inosital that I'd discovered while searching alternative cancer therapy sites on the Internet. I had read about a dog with bone cancer who had received IP-6 and Inosital as part of his treatment plan. I had found it in capsule form at the health food store. Before sprinkling it on Cliff's food, I had tasted the supplement and found it relatively flavorless, so I knew that Cliff would eat it.

I had read some articles indicating that this supplement exhibits some antioxidant functions that have been shown to damage the cells that cause or promote cancer. Its components are naturally occurring substances found in oats, wheat, rice, corn, and legumes. Not only does it suppress the body's production of free radicals, but it also affects the basic mechanisms of cell growth. Unlike conventional cancer treatments, IP-6 and Inosital does not kill cancer cells. Instead, it inhibits cancer by making the cells behave and grow more like healthy cells. Although there were no controlled studies supporting the effectiveness of these kinds of supplements, I felt there was minimal risk, and possibly, a great deal to be gained.

I got the impression that while Dr. Robinson was not familiar with IP-6 and Inosital, she was certainly open to the idea of giving it a try. I also told her that I had accidentally discovered wheat grass juice at a juice bar one day, and that now Cliff, Jokonita, and I were all doing daily shots of it. I had learned that wheat grass juice is thought to be a "blood cleanser," and that it has a detoxifying effect on the body. Cliff and Jokonita seemed to like the taste, and licked each other's bowls after they had finished their own. I guessed that to them, it was similar to chewing grass, as some dogs like to do. Wheat grass juice contains chlorophyll, which is thought to have an effect on the circulatory system and the oxygen supply of the body, in addition to its role in detoxifying and regenerating the liver.

From her warm response to my enthusiasm, I sensed that she understood I was willing to try anything. As she continued the treatment on Cliff, she asked, "Have you ever done Reiki, or worked with an animal communicator?"

"No, I haven't—but I'd be interested in finding out more about both of those things," I said.

She gave me the name and phone number of a woman who did both, Dr. Brenda McClelland, and recommended that I set up an appointment for Cliff right away. I talked a while longer with Narda—we'd achieved first-name familiarity already—discussing the frequency of Cliff's treatments. We were pleased that this first acupuncture session had gone so smoothly. Cliff hadn't seemed to mind the needles at all, and he lay calmly throughout the entire session.

"I'll work with you, and fit you in whenever you're going to be at the VTH," Narda said.

"Thank you so much," I said. "I'll see you on Wednesday, then."

Before she left the room, Narda said, "I'm very interested in knowing what Brenda has to say about Cliff. I also want to make sure you understand—there's a possibility Brenda may tell you some things that you don't really want to hear."

"I feel very sure that Cliff is going to be okay," I said. "I'm not worried about receiving bad news." I truly felt that Cliff would be fine and that we were finally on a path that could heal him.

As I left the VTH that day, I had some new questions. While I was really glad I'd met Narda, and that our first acupuncture session had gone so well, I was still a bit unsure of what to think about Reiki and animal communication. I was willing to keep an open mind, however. When I got back to the hotel, I called Brenda to set up an appointment. She told me that she'd already spoken to Narda, who had filled her in on Cliff's history. We scheduled an appointment for 6:00 P.M. the following day, at the hotel.

The next day, Cliff's chemo treatment went without a glitch. I was happy that we'd started to develop a routine. Since I'd begun sitting with him during his treatments, he would just lay quietly next to me while the chemo drugs were slowly administered. I was a little anxious, because our first appointment with Brenda was to take place that night. I had spent some time on the Internet the night before, reading about Reiki, so I had some idea of what to expect.

I had learned that Reiki is a form of energy work with Japanese origins. It involves sending healing energy to the patient, which the patient's body then uses where it is needed. The practitioner's hands are placed on or over the patient's body. The healing energy flows from the universe, through the practitioner, and into the patient. It works on four levels of the body—physical, mental, emotional, and spiritual. This would be my first experience with a Reiki treatment, and I found the thought of it compelling. I was very interested to see what would actually happen.

In addition, I did some research on animal communication, and was surprised at what I discovered. I learned that Brenda does something that is often referred to as "higher self communication," a phrase that I had never heard before. I quickly learned that the "higher self" is like the subconscious mind. It connects us to all other living things in the world. We don't usually hear what is happening among all of our subconscious ties. However, it *is* possible to communicate with each other this way, usually in times of crisis. One example of this is when a mother hears her child crying in her mind, and knows that her child has been hurt or in an accident. Another example is the way twins often communicate with each other, one twin knowing exactly what the other is doing or feeling, even when they are apart. Brenda uses this technique to convey messages, even from those who cannot speak—our companion animals. I felt intrigued at this thought, and knew that it would be a very interesting experience.

After Cliff's treatment at the VTH, we went back to the hotel. I decided to take Cliff and Nita for a short walk before Cliff's appointment with Brenda. Minutes after we returned, there was a knock at the door. It was Brenda, right on time. Cliff's and Jokonita's ears perked up, and as they started toward the door, I told them to lie down and wait. I opened the door, and Brenda came in. She had long, straight, dark brown hair and was dressed in blue jeans and a sweater. She smiled a bit nervously as she glanced over at Cliff and Jokonita.

"It's okay," I said, as the dogs came over to sniff her. "Won't you sit down?" I said to Brenda. I sat next to her, and told her which dog was which. She reached down to pet them, and we chatted for a few minutes. The dogs quickly found a place on the floor near my feet.

"I have no prior experience with Reiki, or with animal communicators," I said. "Why don't you tell me a bit more?"

Brenda gave me a bit of personal history, and also talked about how she became involved with Reiki and higher self communication. She said that although she sometimes receives images or feelings from the animal, she doesn't rely on this form of communication. Instead, the animal usually responds to her in English.

"When I was a teenager, I began to notice that I had an ability to communicate with animals," Brenda said. "Although I was brought up with more traditional beliefs, I soon realized that I had special skills I couldn't explain." She smiled at me, probably sensing that I was still a little skeptical. Nonetheless, I was very interested in seeing her work on Cliff.

I later found out that Brenda was brought up a Catholic, like I was. She had attended Catholic school through the eighth grade, and then transferred to a public high school. She had attended the University of Southern Colorado and went on to CSU, where she received her doctor of veterinary medicine degree in 1997.

Since Cliff was calmly lying on the floor, Brenda sat down next to him. I watched as she pulled out a crystal on a chain and held it over him. She then moved it up and down over his body. She closed her eyes and sat next to him in total silence. I sat quietly and watched. After a few minutes, she opened her eyes and said quietly, "Cliff does not want to die."

My first thought was, *That's good—I don't want him to die either.*

Brenda said that Cliff told her very clearly that he was going to fight this disease—that he refused to give up.

I watched as she pulled out a book and began to flip through the pages. At one point she stopped, looked at me again, and said, "Wow." Brenda continued to silently communicate with Cliff, naming the flower essences that he needed—tansy, cayenne, mountain pride, and sunflower. I had never used flower essences before, so she explained what they were, where to find them, and how to mix them.

"You should use a glass bottle, four or fives inches tall, with a dropper top," Brenda said. "Then, fill it up three-quarters full with purified water, and add five drops of each flower essence to the bottle. You will need to give Cliff one dropper full, squirting it into his mouth, twice a day, for the rest of his life."

Brenda continued, noting that Cliff needed B vitamins and fish oil, and that we should continue the IP-6 and Inosital and the wheat grass juice. He needed more fiber in his diet, but we should discontinue the bee pollen, as he didn't need it. When she got to the question of homeopathy, she said that he needed Arsenic Album 30x, once a week, for the rest of his life.

I sat there amazed as I watched the session continue. I wondered how it was possible for her to communicate with him. I was a bit skeptical at first, but then I thought to myself, *Who am I to judge?* Just because I didn't know anything about higher self communication prior to this didn't mean it was not possible. There are many powers that people possess, unexplainable powers, and maybe this was just one of them. *What a wonderful gift, to have this ability.*

The session continued for over an hour, and when Brenda finished, I thanked her for coming. "I'll keep in touch with you, and let you know how Cliff is doing," I said.

"Great—I appreciate that. I'll give Narda a call and let her know what I've learned from Cliff today," Brenda said.

Before leaving town the next day, Cliff would receive another acupuncture treatment from Narda at the VTH. I was very eager to see her, and looked forward to hearing her comments about Cliff's session with Brenda. Being naturally curious, I'd done some Internet research on Narda. I needed to get a feel for her background, her training. Did she really believe in the power of Reiki and animal communication? I was very surprised to learn what I did about her.

From the first moment I'd met Narda, I had really liked her. She was very friendly and warm, not too flamboyant, but not too mainstream, either. She had wavy, light-brown hair, slightly longer than shoulder-length. She was very natural looking, and didn't dress like some of the other doctors at the hospital—more like someone I would see at a holistic retreat, wearing Birkenstock sandals. I felt an instant, unexplainable connection to her. I soon learned that she was not only a veterinarian (DVM), but also a doctor of osteopathy (DO). I was very impressed with her credentials and the extensive degrees she held. The fact that she believed in Reiki and animal communication reinforced my conviction that anything was possible.

The next day, I greeted Narda in the treatment room, with Cliff resting calmly nearby. I asked her if she'd had a chance to talk with Brenda.

She grinned. "Yes—and what Brenda told me was very interesting," Narda said. "I should warn you, though, that not all the doctors at the VTH believe in what Brenda does. I think you should take advantage of the information that Brenda gave you, but don't be surprised if you get funny looks when you mention it to others," Narda said.

It was at this moment I decided I really didn't need to tell anyone else about our session with Brenda. I had mentioned it to Kim the day before—that we were going to see Brenda for Reiki—but I hadn't provided any details. I didn't know if Kim was one of those who did not believe. I didn't know who believed and who didn't; in my mind, it didn't really matter. The only thing that mattered was what *I* believed.

We continued with the chemo, acupuncture, and pamidronate once a month for four months. This meant we were spending almost one week a month in Fort Collins and at the VTH, which didn't bother me in the least. The most important thing to me was that Cliff was showing signs of improvement. After the first radiation treatment to the knee, he started to bear more weight on his back leg. I took that as a sign it was not as painful.

Things continued to progress, and each week I saw more and more signs of Cliff's improved mobility. Soon he hardly limped at all, and was able to jump up into the Suburban again. I was pleased to see that he had maintained his appetite, and we never reached a point at which he did not want to eat. He also did not show any signs of nausea, nor did he get diarrhea during these weeks. He became very interested in playing with Jokonita again, and from all outward signs, you would not have known he had cancer. He seemed happy to be alive, and had become more loving and affectionate than ever. It made me wonder how long he had been living with this horrible disease before it became apparent to us.

After the four months of intense treatments, we were finished, except for continuing with the pamidronate and acupuncture on a monthly basis. I asked Kim if this amount of chemotherapy was enough, and she told me that any more was not proven to be helpful—in fact, could even be harmful.

I had become very comfortable with not only Kim, but everyone at the VTH. During the past months, I had come in each day with a smile on my face. I had never shed a tear. I had never second-guessed Cliff's care. I always believed that what we were doing would work. I knew in my heart that Cliff would regain his quality of life. I felt very safe and comfortable there. Long gone were the days when I could not keep my composure. In finding out all that was wrong with Cliff, in a way, we had been granted a new lease on life. I think Cliff felt my positive attitude too. Now that pain was no longer an issue, I saw easier days ahead for us.

Cliff continued to show improvement, and when Jokonita came into heat in the middle of January 2001, I thought, *What the heck? Life is too short. Why not let them have some fun?* And they did mate, multiple times during that week. They ran around the house chasing each other. I felt great joy, and told Kim about it. She felt that Cliff must be feeling well and up to the challenge. It did my heart good to see the life come back into him, and each month things continued to get better. He was regaining muscle mass on his leg, and it was getting stronger. Each month when we went to the VTH, the X-rays and ultrasounds showed no metastasis to any of his organs or lymph nodes. Each time the CBC came back indicating that everything was fine. He was no longer just my inspiration; now, he was inspiring others—the doctors, the staff, and all who met him and heard of his journey. He was my miracle dog.

As winter turned to spring, Cliff continued on the monthly doses of pamidronate and the acupuncture treatments. From all outward signs, it looked like we were winning this battle. Cliff had his mobility back, including full use of his back leg. All of the hair had grown back at the surgery site. The only obvious indication that he'd had cancer was a patch of hair on his back that had lost pigment and turned gray from the radiation to his spine.

The most important thing was the fact he was no longer in pain. His quality of life was as it had been before. That was really all I'd ever wanted for him—to live his final days on this earth being happy and pain-free. Although Kim could not pinpoint which treatment helped him the most, I believed that the pamidronate was a large part of it. It did appear that it was preventing the cancer from spreading throughout the rest of his skeletal system, and I realized then that the work they were doing at the VTH was not only to benefit animals, but to benefit all humankind. These great doctors, both human and veterinary oncologists, were working together with one common goal: to find a cure for cancer, and to find new drugs like the one being used on Cliff. I'd never thought about this much, but cancer is cancer, whether it affects a human or an animal. If a cure can be found for one, it can be used on the other. This gave me renewed hope that they would be successful one day—and perhaps Cliff would play a small role in this important work.

12

Our Return to Pennsylvania—Cliff Romps Again

In April of 2001, we returned to Pennsylvania. Kim coordinated Cliff's monthly pamidronate treatments with my vet in State College, Dr. Alan Friedlander, and on April 12, we had our first appointment with him. We arrived at the Animal Medical Hospital promptly at 10:00 A.M., and were taken to an exam room. Dr. Friedlander came in to talk to us about Cliff's status.

"I've talked to Dr. Selting, and I've been following Cliff's progress over the past few months," Dr. Friedlander said. "I'd like to do a CBC before Cliff starts the treatment, to be sure everything looks good."

I agreed with his plan. I felt comfortable being there, knowing that Kim had gone over everything with him. Cliff and I settled down on a blanket on the exam room floor to wait for the results of the blood work to come back.

In my heart, I knew there was nothing to worry about. During the past few weeks in Pennsylvania, Cliff had been romping and running and chasing the Frisbee again, and it felt good to be back, enjoying the springtime weather. Just the day before, I'd noticed tiny buds popping open on the bushes, and the mountainside above our house was turning a lighter shade of green. I knew that it would only be a matter of weeks until everything was in full bloom, new life growing all around us. It was a great feeling to be able to experience this again with Cliff, to watch as the earth reawakened just as we ourselves, were reawakening. I was more thankful than ever for each breath of air we shared.

Springtime in Pennsylvania had a lot to offer. In addition to the refreshing colors of new grass and flowers, I was also happy to see that my birds were back, visiting the feeder again. It seemed like there was a more colorful variety this year, with lots of jays and cardinals. Maybe they had been there in the past, but I just hadn't seen them. Maybe it was *me* who'd changed during the course of dealing with Cliff's cancer for the past eight months.

Maybe it took a dog to show me what no human could.

As Dr. Friedlander came back to the exam room, my mind returned from its musings. "Cliff's blood work looks great," he said.

"That's great news," I said, feeling relieved, in spite of my confidence that Cliff was okay.

I watched as Dr. Friedlander put on a pair of rubber gloves and placed a mask over his face. Before he took the bottle to mix it with saline, I looked at the label to make sure it was the right drug. He had said that when he ordered it, he had checked and double-checked to be sure it was the same drug they used at VTH. Still, I needed to see for myself.

He took the bottle and went outside to mix it with the saline solution, telling me he was doing it this way to ensure he wouldn't inhale the fumes. Soon he came back with the mixture and hooked it up to the pump. I knew that it would take two hours to complete the treatment. I looked at the pump to see what numbers were displayed; it read the same way that it had at the VTH. I felt good knowing that Dr. Friedlander was following the same procedure Kim had followed.

The catheter they were using was a little shorter than what had been used at the VTH. Because of the way it was positioned in Cliff's vein, every once in a while the alarm beeped, which meant the vein was blocked. I knew what to do, as I'd heard that sound many times during our treatments at the VTH. When this happened, I would just straighten out Cliff's leg a little, and push the start button on the pump to restart it. Over the two hours, this only happened a few times. After my experience at the VTH it had all become second nature to me, and I felt calm and very comfortable being with Cliff during his treatments.

When Dr. Friedlander returned, I smiled up at him from my spot on the floor next to Cliff. I knew the treatment had gone smoothly.

"I'd like a copy of Cliff's blood work for my file," I said to the doctor, "and also, I'd like a copy to be faxed to Dr. Selting." I wanted to ensure that she was still very much involved in Cliff's care. I knew that she had the best team of oncologists working with her, and they had become the foundation that supported me as we continued this battle. Dr. Friedlander said he'd take care of those copies for me, and I thanked him for his help.

After the catheter was disconnected, I quickly took Cliff outside so he could get rid of some of the fluids he'd just taken in. On treatment days, I made sure he had ample opportunity to go out—even in the middle of the night, when we often shared some beautiful moonlit skies. *If it were not for Cliff, I would not have been awake to see them.* These nights together in the outdoors were but one reason why Cliff and I had grown even closer during the past eight months. We had developed a bond that went deeper than anything I'd ever imagined sharing with an animal companion—one of total trust, love, and understanding. I saw those things every time I looked into Cliff's eyes.

A month after our first visit with Dr. Friedlander, we were back at the Animal Medical Hospital for what would be Cliff's last treatment there for a few months. Dr. Friedlander and I chatted a bit about Cliff's progress before he started the treatment. I assumed my usual place on the floor next to Cliff, and the treatment began.

While the medicine was being administered, I allowed my mind to wander, thinking about what we'd experienced, and what lay ahead. We would be leaving for Colorado again soon, and I was very much looking forward to seeing Kim again. I wanted everyone to see Cliff and how well he was doing. They would all be happy to hear he was chasing Jokonita around again.

Two weeks earlier, I'd noticed some drops of blood on the floor, and suspected that Jokonita was coming into heat again. I counted back and realized that her last heat cycle had only been in January. She appeared to be short-cycling, and I suspected this could be part of the reason she had not gotten pregnant the last time. Although I would have loved to have a litter of puppies from her and Cliff, somehow the timing was not right. I wouldn't go to any lengths to keep them apart—if it happened, great—but if not, that would be okay, too. I still had Cliff's sperm banked for future use. I knew that I would need to address Jokonita's apparent infertility eventually, and that I'd need to find a reproduction specialist either here or in Colorado. In reality, though, I was just happy to see that Cliff was still interested.

I thought more about the past few weeks, and other signs that Cliff's quality of life was returning. Amy and Chase had come for a visit recently, and it had been wonderful for them to see how well Cliff was doing. Chase, just a year old, loved Cliff and Jokonita, and whenever he saw them, he would always reach out to touch their fur. Both dogs were very gentle with him when he wrapped his little arms around their necks. They licked his face, and he would smile and giggle. I watched them together and smiled, knowing that I had done the right thing for Cliff. He looked so happy. I knew that one day, the reality of his death would come—if not from cancer, then from something else.

I found this to be one of the great injustices of life—that our beloved animals don't live as long as we do. A small dog's life expectancy is usually less than fifteen years, and a large dog's life is closer to ten years or less, a mere fraction of the average human's life span. I wondered why they were created that way. Was it to humble us? Or perhaps, to underscore the reality of life and death . . . I didn't have the answer. At the very least, I knew I'd done everything in my power to ensure a longer, better life for Cliff. I patted his head as he laid there, the treatment coming to an end.

As I stroked his back, I thought about a recent hike we'd taken. That day, I found myself rejoicing in the fact that Cliff's old gait was back; he was able to walk as he used to, before the cancer. I had been careful not to overdo it on our hikes, while still allowing Cliff the chance to partake in a pastime we had both enjoyed for many years. Even though we no longer took marathon hikes, the joy we shared in being together was never more evident than on this day. I'd found that it wasn't the length of the hike that mattered—it was the quality of the time we spent together. That day on the mountain, I felt that everything we'd gone through had been worthwhile.

Dr. Friedlander returned just as Cliff's treatment came to an end.

"I'll be going back to Colorado soon," I said. "Thank you so much for being here to help us, and to share in Cliff's care." Dr. Friedlander smiled as he rubbed the spot behind Cliff's ears. "When we get back to the VTH," I continued, "they will be doing another bone scan so they can reassess Cliff's condition. I'll be sure to let you know how we make out."

"That's great," the doctor said. "I wish you all the best, and please do keep in touch."

"We will, Dr. Friedlander," I said. As we left, I said good-bye to the staff, telling them we'd see them again in September.

In the meantime, however, we would be returning to the VTH for Cliff's treatments. I realized how far we had come. When I'd spoken to Kim during the past week, she'd mentioned that another dog had come in with bone cancer. Like us, the owners had not wanted to amputate the leg. I remembered when I'd faced that same pivotal moment with Cliff. Although I didn't know what those owners had decided to do for their dog, I was just grateful that the path we'd chosen for Cliff had turned out to be the right one for us.

Another one of the oncologists had recently asked Kim how Cliff had been doing on the pamidronate, and she'd told him of the great success we had experienced. It was a really good feeling to know that others might be helped from our experience. The different treatments we'd tried, the alternative therapies—everything that had worked so well for Cliff might also help other dogs.

Despite my confidence and happiness over the success of Cliff's treatment, the thought of Cliff having another bone scan still scared the hell out of me. But I knew that in reality, whatever was going to show up was going to show up, regardless. It was better to know what we were dealing with than to avoid it. We had done everything we could possibly do with both conventional and unconventional medical treatments, and I felt I'd made good on my promise to try anything that was available to help Cliff.

I had to believe it was helping, as Cliff was thriving.

13
Spondylosis

JULY 2001

It was July 23, and Jokonita and I had just arrived at Boyd Lake. The skies were threatening, and there were a few flashes of lightning in the distance. I had decided that we'd take our chances with the weather, as Nita had been in the car all morning and needed some time to run. I needed some fresh air too.

The morning had been tough on me emotionally. I had dropped Cliff off at the VTH at 10:30 for a bone scan, ultrasound, X-rays, and a CBC. As before, I wouldn't be able to see him until his body had eliminated the radioactive fluids injected for the scan, and being away from him for the next twenty-four hours would be the worst part. It had been great to see Kim, and she was pleased to see how well Cliff was walking. It would be later in the day before she would have the results from the tests, and as usual, she said that I could either call or stop back in. Knowing I had a few hours to kill, I had decided to take Jokonita to the lake for a while.

While I couldn't imagine that Kim would have bad news for me, I couldn't help but feel a little nervous and edgy. I really hated leaving Cliff, and I couldn't get him off my mind. He had been amazing; so wonderful and trusting each time I dropped him off at the VTH. He always went calmly with whoever was there to greet us. I felt sure he understood that they were there to help him—especially since he was no longer experiencing intense pain.

It was one of those days when no one else was at the lake, and I didn't see a single boat out. Although I knew we probably shouldn't be out in this weather either, it was the kind of day when the world's energy felt vibrant and alive. The black clouds raced quickly across the sky. The tumbleweeds rolled in the wind, flying all around us. I quickly zipped up my jacket and pulled up my hood. Jokonita hopped out and we headed right down to the water. Along the way I threw the Frisbee to her. She seemed oblivious to the weather, just happy to be out playing.

After a while, we headed back to the Suburban. I had some errands to do, and decided I'd take Nita along with me. It was too early to check into the hotel yet, so I decided to call Kim to see how things were going.

When the receptionist answered, I told her my name, and asked her to page Dr. Selting. "I think they're still doing rounds, but I'll double-check," she said. After putting me on hold for a minute or so, she came back on the phone and told me that Dr. Selting was still on rounds, but that she'd left a message for me: Cliff's CBC, ultrasound, and X-rays looked great. In addition to the chest X-rays, they had also taken some of Cliff's knee. Kim was pleased to report that the bone in Cliff's knee was remineralizing. They were still waiting for the results of the bone scan.

This was wonderful news! I thanked the receptionist for the message, and breathed a sigh of relief. *So far, so good.*

I ran a few errands, trying to make the time fly by, and at 5:00 P.M. I headed back to the VTH. I brought Cliff's favorite dinner—his usual rotisserie turkey from Boston Market—and would ask Kim to give it to him later. When I got to the VTH, I asked them to page Kim. I took a seat, not knowing how long it would be.

Just a few minutes later, Kim came out to meet me. "The bone scan results are back," she said.

My heartbeat quickened; I couldn't get a word out, and it was hard to interpret Kim's expression.

"All of the sites look the same, or better, with the exception of a site on Cliff's spine, which appears to be larger than it was before," Kim said, her voice shaking slightly.

I was startled, and I could tell that Kim was also unnerved. She proceeded to tell me about two different treatments we should consider:

The first was to have some X-rays taken the next morning, and have the radiologist compare them to the bone scan, as well as to all of the prior X-rays and scans. This would be particularly critical, because they needed to determine how much—if any—radiation this site had already received.

"There's always the potential of damaging the spinal cord when radiating the spine," Kim said. "Doing so could result in neurological damage to Cliff's back end and legs, so we need to be sure that more radiation is our best option."

The second option Kim proposed was a new type of radiation called Samarium-153-EDTMP. It is rarely used, and involves a radioactive isotope taken up in areas that needed bone repair. One problem with this type of treatment is the fact that only two places in the United States were offering this treatment at the time—one in Missouri, and the other in Texas. The big issue with this choice was that Cliff would have to stay in the hospital for five days, because it takes a while for the body to eliminate the radioactive fluids. This meant I would not be allowed contact with him during that entire time. Kim and I both agreed this would not be good for Cliff. We did not want to expose him to any undue suffering caused by being apart from me—especially when there was no guarantee this procedure would even help with Cliff's type of cancer.

"Every day counts when you're dealing with cancer," Kim said. "It may not be worth it for him to be away from you."

I found this comment particularly disturbing, knowing that she dealt with cancer on a daily basis. What did she mean by that? *Was there something she wasn't telling me?*

We continued to discuss our options, and decided we would start with additional X-rays in the morning, to see if more radiation to the spine was even an option. I hated to leave without seeing Cliff, but knew that I had to.

"Cliff's resting comfortably," Kim assured me. "I'll give him his dinner later."

"Thanks so much, Kim," I said. "I'll see you in the morning—and please, tell Cliff that I love him."

I left and headed back to the lake. I didn't want to go to the hotel yet; I needed to be where I could feel Cliff. I watched as the sun set over Horsetooth Mountain, and I longed for him to be there with me.

It was close to 9:00 P.M. when Jokonita and I got to the hotel. I was ready to have a glass of wine and sit down to write my e-mail update to everyone.

I knew it was going to be a rough night.

The next morning when I arrived at the VTH, I saw Kim in the waiting room with her daughter, Madison. They had stopped by on their way to a field trip, to the Ocean Journey aquarium in Denver. We talked about what was going to happen that day. After the X-rays were taken, the radiologists would get together and decide if Cliff could handle more radiation on his spine. Even though I knew Cliff would be in good hands, I hated to see Kim go. I smiled and told them to have fun at the aquarium—we would be fine.

I sat there waiting patiently, watching the minutes tick by and trying to stay calm and positive. A nurse stopped by and said that Radiology had an opening, and they could take Cliff for the X-rays first; we could sit for the pamidronate afterward. I nodded my head, and handed Cliff over to her. Normally I would have left and taken Jokonita to the lake, but I wouldn't be leaving today. I wanted to be there when Radiology was finished.

So I waited.

During the next hour, I learned a lot about the people who were also waiting with their pets. Most of them were there because their dogs had cancer. A man from Los Angeles waited to pick up his yellow Lab, who had had surgery the day before to save his leg. They had removed a cancerous bone and replaced it with one from a cadaver. Gone were the days when

I could not talk about cancer. Gone were the days when I would have avoided talking to them at all. I had come to realize we were all in this together—with dogs of different sizes and breeds, with many different types of cancer.

I sat and talked, and listened, offering words of encouragement and telling them about Cliff and how well he was doing with his treatments. I felt good, being able to share some of what I'd gone through with Cliff. I could tell by the look in their eyes that they were grateful to talk about their own experiences, too.

At 10:15, Karen, a nurse in the oncology department, came out to tell me that Cliff would not be getting any more radiation. She said that the radiologists had looked at all of Cliff's old films, and had compared them to the ones taken today. They'd even had Cliff brought back to them, so they could examine him in person. They determined that the site in question was not a tumor—instead, it was a condition called spondylosis. Although this word was unknown to me, I was simply overjoyed to hear that it was not more cancer. I soon found out that spondylosis is an arthritic-type condition in which the bones of the spine grow together to provide reinforcement to a weak area. This is common in older dogs, and not something that should worry me too much.

Karen took me back to the exam room, where Cliff was very excited to see me. I bent over to hug him. "I love you," I whispered. He lifted his head up and snuggled in against my chest. I held him close and silently thanked God for the news we had just received.

Karen bent down and began to hook up Cliff's catheter to the pump. From the treatment room I called Narda and left a message for her. Cliff was scheduled to have acupuncture when his pamidronate treatment was over, and I wanted to tell her about the spondylosis. I wanted to know if there were any trigger points she could focus on that might help with the condition. She soon called me back and told me she was happy to hear the news, and that she would be in to see us soon.

A few minutes later, Karen stopped back in to check on us, and we chatted for a while about Cliff. She gave me the medicine that Cliff would need for the week: a low dose of morphine and carprofen. I felt very comfortable knowing that Kim had prepared everyone to take care of us in her absence. Karen unhooked Cliff from the pump, and I quickly took him outside.

I saw Narda in the hallway. "I'll be right in to do Cliff's acupuncture," she said.

As she worked on Cliff, I sat on the floor and talked to her about his bone scan, and the scare we'd had with the spondylosis. I was very happy to have her to talk to; she had been a positive influence on us, and I felt fortunate to have her in our lives.

14
One-Year Anniversary

It was the end of August, and I was sitting with Cliff at the VTH while he received the pamidronate. Suddenly, I realized that the next day would be the one-year anniversary of the discovery of the lump. What a long way he'd come since that day. Cliff had become such an inspiration to everyone at the VTH, and when Kim had come to meet us that morning, she'd taken him in the back to show him around. She wanted to be sure that Sue, the critical-care nurse who had cared for him during his overnight visits, could see how well he was doing.

Even though this had been a tiring week for Cliff—with Jokonita in heat again—I could tell he was much stronger as I watched him run after her in the woods like a two-year-old. He was his old self again! True, he had dropped a few pounds, but Kim didn't seem too concerned, since he usually lost weight when Jokonita was in heat. Looking at him, you would never even know that he had cancer. He looked absolutely wonderful.

I glanced up at the monitor on the pump and noticed it read 58, and I knew we only had a short time left. I looked at Cliff, lying on his side, and noticed that he was sleeping. He must have been dreaming, because his legs were twitching ever so gently. As I looked at him, I was overwhelmed with gratitude that he was still alive. I didn't think I could love him more than I did at that moment.

As strange as it might sound, I could communicate with him in a way I never knew was possible. There was something that I simply could not explain. I felt he understood me just as I understood him. It was not a spoken language—more of a silent communication between two very different souls.

Until Cliff had come into my life, I had never known such a bond could exist between a human being and an animal. He had become a part of my heart. Sure, it had been a long, hard year at times, but it had also been a year of intense growth for me. I had allowed my deepest fears to be replaced with hope and faith. As I looked at Cliff, I thought back to what an acquaintance of mine had said about him—that he got cancer so I could learn about real love. At the time, I'd thought it rather a silly notion, but in hindsight, I realized that this was exactly what had happened. Not that Cliff had chosen to get cancer, but possibly, that the path had been chosen for us—so we could share the experience, and learn and grow from it.

My mind started to drift, remembering things from my childhood, things I thought I'd buried long ago.

My mother had died when I was sixteen, and from that day on I had created my own world to live in. Without realizing it, I had put up walls to keep out that kind of pain. The morning she died, I'd heard a thump downstairs, but had stayed in my bedroom for a few minutes before going down to check it out. When I did, I found her lying on the floor, not breathing.

Sometimes I wondered what I had missed by not having her in my life for the last twenty-four years. How would my life have been different? What type of person would I have become if I hadn't had to face those early challenges? I'd never had a chance to save her, but now, with Cliff, I had been given that opportunity.

Maybe Cliff had been sent to help me let it go—to help me believe in miracles. He had made me care so deeply for him that I was willing to try anything to save him. I had taken a risk, allowing pain to enter into my heart again, and in so doing, I had found a very different type of love. I had learned to experience life though a dog's eyes. Whether it was the hikes we took together or the sunsets we watched, or the quiet times, like this moment, as I watched the drugs dripping into his veins. Loving Cliff so deeply had set me free.

Kim would be back soon; she had gone to get Cliff's medications for me. That morning we'd been discussing what we thought Cliff needed for pain. He was still on one extended-release morphine pill per day, and one carprofen. Kim had said the pamidronate was known to help with pain in humans who had bone cancer, but we really had no way of judging the extent of the pain animals experienced, except by taking them off the medications to see how they did without them. I did not want Cliff to be in any pain, so I told her I would like to keep him on the low dose of morphine for now. As for the carprofen, Kim advised that we keep him on it, as well. It would help with any pain he might have from the spondylosis.

As Kim opened the door a few minutes later, Cliff stirred and lifted his head to see who was there. She smiled at us and asked how Cliff was doing. "Fine," I said, as she sat down on the floor next to us. I was very happy she was there. If only she knew what I had been thinking about—how my life had been forever changed by Cliff and his cancer. *One day I will tell her.* I believed that she had been our savior, sent to help Cliff and me. She was more than Cliff's doctor; she was also my friend, and I knew she would always be an important part of our lives.

Kim unhooked the catheter from Cliff and reached into her white coat pocket, pulling out a written prescription for the morphine, which could be filled at any pharmacy. "The carprofen will be at the pharmacy window here, and you can pick it up on your way out," Kim said.

"Okay—that's great," I said. "We're going to leave town right away, so I can miss the Denver rush-hour traffic."

Kim gave Cliff a hug, and then stood up and gave me one, too.

"I'll stay in touch once we get back to Pennsylvania," I said. We were leaving in a few days. "But I'll back in October, and we'll see you then."

It was hard for me to leave the VTH sometimes. I wondered if Kim had any idea how grateful I was. She and her colleagues were just doing their jobs, trying to help animals who had cancer, but what they were really doing was making this world a better place. They showed us kindness and compassion. They were human angels who walked this earth, caring for our beloved animal companions—God's real gift to humankind, and to me.

I had been so deeply involved in Cliff's struggle with cancer that there hadn't been much room for any other distractions in my life. Little did I know that on September 11, 2001, our world would be changed forever, our entire country plunged into a nightmare beyond comprehension.

I will never forget that morning. While the world as we knew it was crumbling, my friend Kate and I were riding our bikes on a beautiful country road in rural Pennsylvania. Upon ending our ride, Kate and I stopped at a local health food store for a snack. That was when we first heard the news.

In a state of shock, Kate and I rushed home. During the drive back, I listened to the horrific radio accounts of what had happened—not only in New York City and Washington, D.C., but also in the small rural area of Shanksville, Pennsylvania. How was it possible that as I was enjoying this beautiful fall day filled with blue skies and sunshine, so many lives had been lost in a place only a few hours away?

When I got home, I was lovingly greeted at the back gate by Cliff and Jokonita. I walked into the backyard and sat down on the deck steps. Cliff sat down on one side of me and Nita on the other. Cliff's eyes were fixated on me, and I sensed he did not understand why I was so upset. As I sat there with tears running down my face, Cliff snuggled in closer to me. I reached down and put an arm around each of them, thankful for the comfort they silently provided.

Why is it, I wondered, *that more humans don't possess the qualities that dogs do?* Dogs don't deceive; dogs don't hate; dogs are not vengeful. Dogs provide love and comfort, strength and kindness. If we were all to practice what we learned from dogs, the world would be a much kinder place.

In October, we came back to Colorado for Cliff's treatment, after being in Pennsylvania for a month. The events of 9/11 had greatly impacted air travel, and I felt extremely fortunate to have access to a private plane. Although security measures had been tightened for all types of aircraft, being able to fly in a private plane made traveling less stressful.

Cliff continued to do well, but I'd noticed a few weeks before that once again, he had started straining when he was trying to relieve himself. I knew that I would be seeing Kim, so I wanted to have her check him out to be sure no cancer had returned to the original site. Even though extensive radiation had been done on his anal gland, there was still a chance that a cancer cell could have survived.

It took us a little longer to get to the VTH this time. Though it was only October, it was snowing over the Vail Pass, and the roads were very slippery. I called Kim on the way to let her know we might be a little late.

"Don't worry about it," she said. "Just have them page me when you arrive."

I was looking forward to seeing her, and having her examine Cliff. It had been a month since our last visit, and I wanted her to reassure me that everything was okay. When we got there, they paged Kim, and she quickly came out to see us.

"Cliff looks great," she said enthusiastically. "I'd like to just take him back to one of the exam rooms and do a rectal exam, to see if everything feels the same as it did the last time." After being gone for only a few minutes, she brought him back out to me, saying she didn't feel anything unusual. But since I'd noticed him straining lately, she thought it prudent to do some X-rays, to make sure we weren't overlooking anything.

"I've already drawn the blood for the CBC and the BUN," Kim said. His BUN had been a little high lately, and she wanted to continue to keep an eye on it to make sure that his kidneys were functioning properly.

After one of the X-ray technicians came to get Cliff, once again I found myself sitting in the waiting room, watching the people with their dogs and cats come and go, knowing all too well that most of them were there for the same reason I was. Sooner than I expected, I saw Cliff pulling the X-ray technician down the hall, trying his best to get to me as fast as he could. *That's Cliff, my baby, my angel.* Cancer could not take away his zest for life.

A few minutes later, Kim came over and sat down next to us. "His X-rays look fine, and his BUN is okay too," Kim said. "His prostate is a little enlarged, and that could be what's causing him the problem; it may be putting pressure on his colon. We should keep an eye on it and, if need be, we can have him neutered, which will allow the prostate to shrink. This is similar to what happens to human males, who tend to have enlarged prostates as they age."

Cliff was approaching the age of ten, so we decided to keep an eye on it, and if he needed surgery in the future, we would do it.

"I've started giving Cliff stool softeners, and they seem to be helping," I said.

"Keep on doing that," Kim said, nodding her approval. "I'd like to take Cliff in the back again and have Dr. Withrow do a rectal exam on him, just to make sure I haven't missed anything." A few minutes later, Kim came back and said that Dr. Withrow hadn't felt anything unusual either.

"Cliff's becoming quite a success story," Kim said, smiling. "I'm glad that I've been able to play a part in his care."

"Thank you so much for your kind words," I said with a heartfelt grin. "That means a lot to me."

A short time later, Dr. Withrow saw us in the waiting room and stopped by to say hello. "Keep up the good work," he said warmly, "and continue whatever you've been doing for Cliff."

I smiled to myself. *I wonder if he knows about all of the alternative therapies I've been using . . . and if he'd believe, as I do, that they've been helping?*

Before leaving, I told Kim that I was going back to Pennsylvania for a while, and would have Cliff's next treatment done there. I'd see her when I returned to Colorado in December. We hugged, and promised to stay in touch.

Cliff and I turned and walked out the door. I felt that all was well.

15
A Turn of Events

New Year's Eve of 2001 found me sitting with Cliff in the critical care unit of the VTH. There were two pumps clamped to the railing overhead, and tubes hanging every which way from the five bags filled with various fluids, all connected to Cliff. There was also a bag attached to him, slowly filling with dark-yellow urine. Kim had been in earlier to visit him, and said she was happy to see that the urine had a concentrated appearance to it. Cliff seemed to be resting comfortably, and was falling into a deep sleep.

The past four days had been extremely difficult for Cliff. I'd brought him back to the VTH on December 27, and his condition had only gotten worse since then. It was hard to believe that only eight weeks had passed since our last visit to the VTH—and that things had shifted so drastically in that brief period of time.

I'd known something was wrong ever since we'd returned to Colorado on December 21. Cliff just hadn't been himself. The vomiting had started on the twenty-third, and continued into the twenty-fourth. On the morning of that day, I'd taken him in to see Dr. Warren, our vet in Edwards, Colorado, who gave Cliff some intravenous fluids and some medicine to help calm his stomach. That night, I picked him up at 6:00, and he appeared to be feeling much better after the fluids.

It was very short-lived. After being home and feeling better on Christmas Eve and Christmas Day, he was soon vomiting again. On the twenty-sixth, I took him back down to see Dr. Warren, who again gave him fluids and also took some abdominal X-rays. I left for a short time while he was getting the fluids, and called at 1:30 P.M. to check on him. A nurse answered the phone, and I could sense from her tone that the news was not going to be good.

"Dr. Warren would like you to come back as soon as possible," she said. "The doctor will go over everything when you get here."

When I arrived, Dr. Warren looked concerned. "I think Cliff has either an ulcer, or possibly a tumor on the wall of his stomach," he said. "I see a spot on the X-ray that doesn't look right."

I picked up my cell phone and immediately called the VTH. I asked to speak with Kim, but was told she was off that week, on Christmas vacation. I asked who was there, hoping for a familiar name—someone who knew Cliff's case. As it turned out, most of the doctors I knew, and those who had seen Cliff in the past, were also off that week. Not knowing what to do next, I asked to speak to Dr. Withrow. I was put through to his voice mail, where I left a very detailed message explaining what was going on with Cliff. Right after I'd finished leaving my message for Dr. Withrow, my cell phone rang. Kim was on the other end.

"I was at the VTH checking my messages," she said. "I just heard your message from a few days ago, about Cliff being sick."

"I'm so happy to hear your voice," I said. I told her what was going on, and passed the phone to Dr. Warren so he could explain what he was seeing on the X-rays. After speaking to Dr. Warren, Kim talked to me about the next step. We decided that I would go to the VTH the next morning. "We'll check Cliff out and scope his stomach for cancer," she said, pausing for a moment as she waited for my reply.

"Okay," I said. Somehow I couldn't think of anything else to say, as the word *cancer* echoed in my ears.

I took Cliff home. It was a long night.

On the morning of December 27, I packed a few things and said good-bye to my family. Amy, Andy, Chase, and Blake were there, visiting for the Christmas holiday. Dick offered to go with me to the VTH, but I said, "No, you stay here with them. I'll take Cliff and Jokonita with me." I needed to be there for Cliff, and I did not want any distractions.

When I got there, I met Dr. Withrow, and the first thing he said to me was, "Cliff looks quite different from the last time I saw him—just eight weeks ago." I nodded, feeling suddenly cold.

"The first thing I want to do is a CBC, to compare it to the one that Dr. Warren recently did," Dr. Withrow said. In addition, he wanted to do a serum chemistry profile and a urinalysis. Later, when the results came back, I knew they weren't good.

"I'm concerned because Cliff's calcium is very high," he said. "I'm worried about Cliff's kidneys, and the possibility of kidney failure."

Dr. Withrow introduced me to another doctor, Dr. Greg Ogilvie, and told me that Dr. Ogilvie would be taking over Cliff's care from this point on. I was somewhat surprised to hear this, as I had never even met him before this moment. Dr. Ogilvie was of average height, with a very thin build. He had a thick mustache, and his dark hair was thinning a little on the top. My first impression of Dr. Ogilvie was that he was very straightforward and to the point. While he didn't sugarcoat anything, he spoke with kindness, and he filled me with a sense of calm.

I soon found out that Dr. Ogilvie knew Cliff well; in fact, he'd been the one behind Cliff's care all along. I later learned that Dr. Ogilvie was the board-certified oncologist who had trained Kim, and the boss she'd referred to in the past. Kim reported to Dr. Ogilvie, since she was still an oncology resident. I was thankful he was there to help us now. Since I now knew he was familiar with Cliff's case, I put my trust in him right away.

"I need to take some new X-rays so I can get an idea of what's going wrong with Cliff's body," Dr. Ogilvie said. "You can wait here in the exam room; I'll be back shortly."

A short while later, he came back in the room, walked over to the exam table, and started to write on a note card all of the things that were wrong with Cliff. He went over them with me: kidney damage, high serum calcium, nodules in lung, mass on kidney, small liver. He turned the note card over and drew a picture as he tried to explain to me the nodules in Cliff's lungs. I stood there in total shock. *Only a week ago, Cliff was running and playing with Nita.* Dr. Ogilvie showed me the X-rays and compared them to the ones that Dr. Warren had taken just a few days before. He also compared them to the ones last taken in Pennsylvania—but most important, to the ones that were taken at the VTH, just eight weeks ago. What he was seeing on Cliff's lungs was new; it wasn't there the last time.

"Where has Cliff been lately?" asked Dr. Ogilvie. "There's a slight chance this could be some type of fungal disease. It's only found in certain parts of the country," Dr. Ogilvie said. That gave me a glimmer of hope.

I tried to grasp everything Dr. Ogilvie was telling me, including the fact that our first problem was Cliff's kidneys. "There's a chance that if the damage to them is recent, it can possibly be reversed," Dr. Ogilvie said. My first thought was, *Finally—something positive.* I simply didn't understand how things could have changed so quickly, from only a week ago.

"How could this happen so fast?" I asked, unable to stop the quaver in my voice.

Dr. Ogilvie looked me straight in the eye and said, "That's how cancer works. It just reappears for whatever unknown reason." He paused for a moment, and then said, "I'm going to take Cliff to the critical care unit. Once we get him started on fluids, I'll come and find you."

During all of this, Cliff had been sitting next to me; I could see how weak he was becoming, right before my eyes. He had lost weight over the past few days, and seemed tired and lethargic. Dr. Ogilvie hadn't given me much hope, saying that it was likely Cliff would die from his disease. I bit my lip and tried to choke back the tears. As he turned to take Cliff to CCU, Dr. Ogilvie put his hand on my shoulder. "I'm sorry," he said simply.

I walked outside. Jokonita was in the Suburban, and I didn't want her to see me cry. I sat down on the grass, away from the car, and then I cried—sixteen months' worth of tears. I sat there for the entire hour it took before Dr. Ogilvie came outside to find me. I just looked at him while I tried to regain my composure. Here I was, facing a man I had just met, clinging to the hope that he could save Cliff. He was our last hope, and I was not ready to give up yet.

"Do you want to go to the CCU and sit with Cliff?" he asked gently.

"Yes," I said, still trying to steady my voice. When I got there, I found Cliff hooked up to the tubes and monitors. His ears perked up when he saw me, and I knew I was where I needed to be. Cliff was in a huge concrete run with wire sides, and many soft blankets for a bed. I went inside the run and sat in the corner, next to Cliff. I sat there in silence, hugging him and willing him to be well again.

Dr. Ogilvie called Kim at home, and she came in to see us. I had a hard time holding back my tears when I saw her, but I was trying to stay strong for Cliff. As I was sitting there, I showed Kim a few tiny lumps on Cliff's head that I had just noticed a few days before. She went to find Dr. Ogilvie, and I watched as they shaved the spot around one of the lumps, numbed it, and removed it. Dr. Ogilvie quickly took it to the lab as Kim stapled shut the incision area. They would have the results back in the morning.

I stayed with Cliff for a while longer, but I knew I had to leave soon because Jokonita was waiting for me in the Suburban. Cliff seemed to be resting comfortably, so I let myself out. I found Dr. Ogilvie down the hall. "I'll be back first thing in the morning," I said. "I need to leave now, to take care of Jokonita."

"Someone will be with Cliff in CCU all night," Dr. Ogilvie said. "If you want to call to check on him, you can."

I left and went back to the hotel with Jokonita. I moved around numbly, giving her food, taking her out when she needed to go. I felt like I was moving in slow motion, through a thick fog.

I finally called Dick. I told him that Cliff was in CCU and they were giving him fluids to try to improve his kidney functions. I did not tell him how bad they feared it was, or that Dr. Ogilvie had told me Cliff could die from his disease. This was something I was not yet willing to accept.

A few hours later, I called CCU to see how Cliff was doing, and was told that he was resting comfortably.

I had a very restless night; everything Dr. Ogilvie had told me was rolling around in my head. A thought came to me about fungal disease. We'd had a very wet fall in Pennsylvania, and there were lots of mushrooms growing in the woods. *Could they have caused the nodules in Cliff's lungs?*

I couldn't sleep, so I got out of bed and found the card Dr. Ogilvie had given me with his number on it. Even though it was 3:15 A.M., I figured I could leave him a message. I also called Kim's office and left her the same message, hoping that the two of them would confer before I saw them the next morning. This brought me a small bit of peace, and I was finally able to get some rest.

On December 28, I woke up at 6:45 A.M. and saw that I had a message on my cell phone. It was from Dr. Ogilvie—Greg, as we were already on a first-name basis with each other. He had received my message, but unfortunately, the type of fungal disease he'd been referring to had nothing to do with mushrooms. He said that Cliff was still comfortable, and that the lab reports would be back by late morning. He would know more then. I called him back and said I'd be in to see Cliff as soon as I could get Jokonita taken care of; she'd had a restless night, too, and was probably wondering what was going on with Cliff.

When I arrived at the VTH, I found Greg right away. He did not have good news for me. We walked back to be with Cliff. "I was hoping that Cliff's condition would have improved from being on the fluids," Greg said, "but he's actually gotten slightly worse. In spite of giving Cliff the fluids, his kidneys are just not improving."

"Can I take him outside to see Jokonita?" I asked.

Greg said that would be okay. Cliff was too weak to walk very well on his own, so Greg asked a technician to help me take Cliff outside. I put a blanket on the ground and the three of us sat down on it. Jokonita was very happy to see Cliff, and as she sniffed him and licked his head, he did the same to her. It was a cool December day, but the sun was out, and it felt good to be outside with them. We sat there for a while, until Greg came out to find us. He brought along the same technician who had helped Cliff outside.

"I want to take Cliff back to CCU so they can get him back on the fluids," Greg said. I nodded, and we walked back in together. Greg asked me to sit down so we could talk. Ironically enough, we ended up sitting in the same seats where I'd often sat while waiting for Cliff to come back after his treatments. Greg looked at me intently.

"What do you want for Cliff?" he asked.

I was struggling to fight back the tears as I looked at him. "What I want, you can't give me." I don't think he was prepared to hear this, and we were both quiet for a few seconds.

"What do you want for Cliff's quality of life?" he asked.

I remained quiet.

He explained the option of euthanizing him. I looked at him and said no. "Cliff will let me know when it's time for him to leave," I said. "We are not giving up yet—not as long as there's a sparkle in his eye."

Greg said, "Okay. That decision is yours to make."

After following Greg back to CCU, I sat there staring at Cliff and thinking that if we could just get his kidneys to function again, there was hope. I knew that as long as Cliff was not in pain, I was making the right choice.

A little while later, Greg came in and said the lab results were back. "The lump we biopsied yesterday is cancer," Greg said. "Knowing that, I'm pretty sure what we're seeing in Cliff's lungs is cancer too." For once, Greg didn't look me in the eye.

I could find no words. I just sat there, staring into space.

Greg left, but came back in a few minutes, hunching down next to me with a box of tissues in his hand. I could no longer deny the fate that lay ahead for Cliff. Greg sat there with us for a little while, and I found comfort in his presence, his warmth and kindness. A couple of times, he tried to make small talk, asking me why we'd decided to move to Colorado. He seemed to understand when I could barely respond. Although we were just getting to know each other, I found that I was starting to rely on him.

Maybe this was the final twist of fate: *I would have to learn to trust a total stranger to care for Cliff during his last days on this earth.*

The next two days, December 29 and 30, were pretty much the same, and I spent most of the time sitting in the CCU with Cliff. Not much had changed; he was still hanging on. Although still hooked up to multiple machines, he was very alert. We were at the point where they were measuring Cliff's "ins and outs"—in other words, measuring the amount of fluids he took in compared to the amount he put out. I tried to get him to drink a little water, just enough to wet his palate. Because he was getting fluids intravenously, I wasn't too concerned when he didn't seem to want any. Greg wanted to keep strict track of his "ins," so I was sure to let them know how much Cliff was drinking.

At one point during the day of December 31, Greg came to sit with us, and I told him that I'd secretly started giving Cliff some herbs to help his kidneys. I felt like I had to be totally honest with him.

"What are you giving him?" he asked. I showed him the bottle.

"I don't think they will help at this point," he said, "but neither will they hurt."

Cliff didn't like them, and I couldn't blame him, since I'd tasted them and thought they were pretty nasty. So I tried rubbing them onto his body, just hoping that they would somehow be absorbed into his system, and by some miracle, help him during this struggle. It had been sixteen months now, and I had seen a lot of small miracles along the way. I had no reason to believe there wasn't one more out there for us.

Greg left again, but came back a short while later. I could tell he was running out of things to say to me. It was obvious he was trying to prepare me for the worst, but I was still not listening. What happened next surprised even me. Greg was sitting next to Cliff, and I asked him, "If Cliff makes it to tomorrow, to January first, will he have a better chance of surviving?" I had heard that more people and animals die at the end of the year than any other time. It was said this was because the light on the other side is strongest at the end of the year—that dying souls are being pulled toward that light. Here it was, December 31, and I needed to know what Greg believed.

"Yes, we do tend to lose more patients at the end of the year," Greg said. "That seems to be the trend. However," he said, looking at me seriously, "I don't think that making it until tomorrow would save Cliff's life."

I knew then that he believed the end was near, although he didn't put it that way. He left us, and I sat there thinking about what we had just discussed. I did not know what to believe; I merely wanted Cliff to live.

A short while later, Kim came to see us. Greg had probably been talking with her, as she said she needed to speak with me. "It's only going to be a matter of time now until Cliff dies," she said softly, her voice breaking. "I want to know what you would like for Cliff." We talked about CPR, and I said that if it came to that, to not do it, because it would be his time to go.

"Cliff could die at any time now," Kim said again, "even when you're outside taking care of Jokonita, or in the bathroom."

I looked at her solemnly, and said, "No. He won't do that. He won't die without me here."

She didn't know what to say to that. I saw the tears well up in her eyes. She left us a short while later, saying that Greg would be gone from the hospital for a little while—he was taking his daughter to see *Harry Potter and the Sorcerer's Stone*.

"I'll be fine here with Cliff," I said. "If there's anything I need, I'll find you."

I sat there thinking about what she'd said, still feeling in my heart what I knew to be true. *Cliff would not die without me there.*

About an hour had passed, and Cliff was lying with his head on my lap, staring into my face. I looked down at him, into his deep, dark brown eyes. Without planning to, I said to him, "It's okay . . . you can go now." Cliff took one final stretch, and I felt the breath leave his body. I knew then that he had left me, and was now in a world where I could not reach him. I knew he was in a place of peace.

One of the technicians must have heard the monitor beep when Cliff's heart stopped. She rushed over to me, saying frantically, "He's gone."

"I know," I said, surprisingly calm. "It's okay. I need Kim."

Kim came to me as I sat there quietly with Cliff, stroking his head and telling him that I loved him, that I was proud of him. She knew that I wanted an autopsy done, something I'd discussed with Greg. Cliff's remains would be cremated, and she told me she would take care of that for me. She also said she would call Greg to let him know that Cliff had passed peacefully.

Kim turned to leave as I continued stroking Cliff's head. "Take as much time as you need," she said softly.

She came back a few minutes later with a pair of scissors, cutting a lock of his hair for me to keep. She then made a mold of his right front paw for me to take with me. I sat there for a while, knowing that when I left, it would be the last time I would ever see Cliff's body. I did not want to leave him, even though I knew he was already gone. I wondered if he could see me from where he was now. Could he see me sitting there, holding his body, loving him until the very end? I felt a very calm sense of peace, and I knew that he was still with me. No longer in the physical world, but still with me and still very much alive in my heart. I finally managed to make my way out of there, taking one last look at Cliff's lifeless body before leaving. He looked peaceful, and for that, I was glad. I wanted to see Greg before I left, but I didn't know if he was back yet. I decided to call his office, leaving a message there to thank him, and to let him know his work was now done. I did not know what else to say, or how to say it. He tried until the very end to save Cliff's life, but in the end, it was out of our hands.

As I was pulling out of the parking lot, the song playing on the radio was "Spirit in the Sky." This wasn't a coincidence, I thought. This was Cliff's way of reaching out to me from the world he was now in. I called Dick and told him that Jokonita and I would be home in a few hours, and that Cliff was now in heaven. On the way home I received a call from Greg. I didn't pick up the call, but let it go to my voice mail. I didn't know what to say to him, to the man I'd never really known, the man I now would never forget. I'd only met him five days before, but in that time I had shared with him some of the most precious moments of my life—my final moments with Cliff. I knew that I could never thank him enough for trying to save Cliff's life. I knew that I would feel a connection to him forever.

When I got home, Dick met me at the door. Amy, Andy, Chase, and Blake were all there too. All I wanted to do was go to bed. I was beyond drained. I went into my bedroom and lay down on the bed. I had brought Cliff's purple fleece blanket back from the VTH, and I spread it over me, trying to find his scent.

"What can I do for you?" Dick asked.

"Nothing," I said. There was nothing that anyone could do for me.

He left and came back with a glass of wine, setting it on the nightstand. I drank it, hoping it would help to numb the pain. A little while later he came back in again and sat down on the bed. I was crying, curled up into a ball. He put his arms around me and said, "It's okay. My dad is taking Cliff for a walk now."

I cried harder, but was grateful for his attempt to comfort me. It was New Year's Eve, a day of celebration, the day before our wedding anniversary. I lay there for a few hours, unable to sleep. After I knew everyone was in bed, I decided to get up and let the many friends and family who had given us support during this battle know of Cliff's passing. I went to my computer and sent out the following e-mail:

To all of you who have been there for the last sixteen months . . .

Today Cliff's battle ended. It came on quickly; only nine days ago he started showing signs of not feeling well. The end was quick and swift, and I am sure it was Cliff's way of protecting me, as he always has. I am thankful that I was with Cliff's doctors at CSU for the last few days. They were there to guide me, to help both Cliff and me, and most importantly, to listen. They were not judgmental, nor did they try to sway me when I decided I wanted to let Cliff tell me when he was ready to go.

It was a tough battle, but one that we won. We got an extra year that no one ever thought we would have. It was a great year, and for the most part, Cliff's life was filled with more good than bad. He enjoyed his life, and I enjoyed him. It was quick today; he was in no pain, just tired, and although he was still fighting, the fight was over. As I lay with him, his head on my lap and my arms around him, I looked down at him, and his big brown eyes were looking up at me, and at that moment, I told him that it was okay, that he could go. He stretched, took a deep breath, and I felt his soul leave his body and a great sense of peace. It was a truly unbelievable experience, one that I will never forget.

I stayed with him for a while, holding him, stroking his head, talking to him and telling him that I loved him, and that I was happy he had been a part of my life. That I was proud of him, and even though he was in a different world now, he would always live on in my heart. His soul was now part of mine, and the years that I had with him taught me about love, unconditional love. The type of love where no matter how many times I took him to the hospital for treatments, no matter how many pills I forced down him, he still yelped with joy every time he saw me. He was truly my soul mate.

Kim was right next door when it happened, and brought over a mold and made a print of Cliff's right paw. I clipped locks of his hair, and brought home with me all the things that were with him in the end. Thank you,

Steve, Kim, Greg, and all the nurses and staff of Critical Care for being there the last few days, and making the unbearable, bearable.

I am home now and miss Cliff dearly. I can still smell him on my shirt, and so does Jokonita. She is wondering where her buddy is. I know in my heart that I will see Cliff again. When I left the hospital today the song on the radio was "Spirit in the Sky." How appropriate. I know Cliff is now looking down on me, my new Guardian Angel. Please don't mourn for us, but be joyful in knowing that Cliff is at peace, and with that, I shall be too. In the next few months I hope to finish the story of our journey; you will each get a copy. It can be finished now, as Cliff wrote the final chapter. My deepest thanks to all of you . . . for your prayers, your well wishes, your medical expertise, your e-mails, your phone calls, your kindness, your friendship, your understanding— and most of all, for your love.

Because without love, life is meaningless.

Love,
JoAnne, Cliff, and Jokonita

16

Bringing Cliff Home

It had been a little over a week since Cliff had passed away, and I could no longer avoid or deny what I needed to do: I had to go to Fort Collins to bring home Cliff's remains.

His presence had been with me since his last breath. I felt him everywhere, especially when I was on the mountain behind our house. The weather was not great when Jokonita and I started out, and we ran into snow on Vail Pass. The roads were slippery, so I slowed down and took my time.

I had Cliff's purple fleece blanket with me. I took it with me everywhere I went. It was the first thing that touched my skin at night. I couldn't bring myself to wash it, as it was the last thing that had touched him. I missed him so badly that my heart ached. I knew he was at peace, but that didn't fill the void. Kim and Greg had assured me that over time, the pain would lessen. I was looking forward to seeing them after I had picked up Cliff's remains.

The bag with Cliff's things from his last days still sat unpacked in the closet—his brass choker collar, his green Frisbee and water bottle, the newspaper I was reading, the herbs, his treats. Above the bag, I'd hung another fleece blanket he had slept on at the VTH, this one brown. It still smelled like him and had some of his hair on it. Jokonita had been going to it and sniffing it, wondering where he was. She had not seen him since the day we all sat together outside the VTH. If I had known he was going to die when he did, I would have brought her in to see him first.

It had all happened so fast. I had still been clinging to the hope of another miracle that day. I had not planned to say those words to Cliff— it had just happened. I had not expected him to die in my arms like that.

125

He had been waiting for permission to leave me.

When I got to Denver, I called the Precious Memories crematory, where Cliff's body had been taken. Kim had made all the arrangements, and had called me to tell me that I could pick him up. The woman who answered the phone at the crematory put me on hold while she looked for Cliff. She came back and said, "Yes, he's there, sitting on the TV." Her nonchalant attitude kind of broke the ice, and I felt a little more at ease. I asked her what his ashes were in, and she said, "The standard floral box, with a rose on top. Most people are very happy with it."

When I arrived at the crematory, I was surprised at how pretty the property was. Located on the outskirts of Fort Collins, it was surrounded by farmland. It was a very peaceful place. I went inside, and the woman I talked to told me that Cliff was ready to go home. She handed the floral box to me, and I tightly held it in my arms. Not knowing what to say, I just stood there. She asked me if I had any other dogs.

"Yes, I have another German shepherd, Jokonita, who's waiting in the car."

"It's okay to let her out to run around in the yard," she said kindly.

"Thank you," I said, as I gave her the payment. I walked outside, carrying Cliff in my arms. I put him on the front seat and let Jokonita out. We walked around the yard, and I noticed there were tombstones in the ground. I realized then that this was also a pet cemetery. I read the tombstones and knew that a lot of love was buried beneath that ground. I knew that I was not alone—that there were many others like me, grieving the loss of their best friends. I put Jokonita back in the Suburban and grabbed a photo of Cliff from the glove compartment, bringing it inside for the woman to see. I wanted her to see him when he was full of life. I felt very proud to be his mom. She offered her condolences, and I thanked her for taking good care of him.

I left and headed to the VTH to see Kim and Greg. I knew this would be very emotional. They had been supporting me with phone calls and e-mails, but this was the first time I would see them since Cliff's death, just nine days before. I walked up to the desk and asked the receptionist to page Kim—that she was expecting me.

"I haven't seen you for a while," the woman said.

I wanted to say that I'd been there over the holidays, but I couldn't get the words out. "I'll be outside," I told her. "Kim can find me there." I had to get out of the building.

When Kim came outside, we both half smiled, and she gave me a hug. "Do you have Cliff with you?" she asked.

"Yes, I do."

"Greg will be out soon," Kim said.

I knew it would be even harder to see him. I hadn't seen him at all since before Cliff died. A few minutes later, Greg came over to where we were standing. He reached out to hug me, and the tears started running down my face. I couldn't say anything; I just stood there and cried. They both tried to comfort me, but there was nothing they could do to ease my pain.

"Don't rush it," Kim said as she rubbed my back soothingly. "Just take it a day at a time." After a moment, she went on. "We have a support group for people who've lost their pets. You might want to consider it."

"I'm not ready to talk to anyone about it," I said, through my tears.

"That's fine," Kim said, "but I want you to know that they're available. They'll be ready to help if you need them."

I could tell they were having a hard time holding back their own tears. We were all feeling the loss of Cliff. I had to leave, and told them that I would stay in touch. I knew that part of me wanted to stay there all day with them, but eventually, I would have to face the reality of leaving. I didn't know when I would see them again. I was leaving with Cliff, and leaving behind the support and kindness that had helped me get through the past sixteen months. I said good-bye and gave each of them a hug. Greg urged me to be careful driving home, and I assured him that I would.

I had a lot of time for reflection on the drive home, of all that Cliff and I had shared. I'd never thought it would come to this day. I had never imagined that Cliff would be in a pretty floral box, sitting there with me. I laid his purple fleece blanket on my lap and put him on top of it for the drive home. I had to pull over a few times because of the tears blurring my vision. Jokonita knew I was upset, and instead of lying in the back where she normally did, she rode home sitting with her head between the front seats. I was glad she was there.

At one point when I stopped, I pulled out the e-mails that I had received from Greg and Kim after Cliff died. I reread them. I needed their support. I was reaching out for any ounce of comfort I could find.

Dear JoAnne,

Thank you for this lovely e-mail. Your words so beautifully capture so much about Cliff. Thank you. We will miss this gentle creature whose eyes sparkled each time he saw you. Even in these last days, when he saw you, his ears would stand straight up, his eyes would focus so precisely on your face, and his expression was one of joy in seeing you, love in being your best friend and soul mate. I will miss this gentle friend, and you. Please take care of yourself in these difficult days ahead without Cliff. Know that we, and especially Kim and I, stand ready to help you in any way possible, if and when you need us. Expect the many days, weeks, and months to have some moments of missing Cliff, but you won't be alone. We will miss him too, and you. We look forward to your book about Cliff. If you do have a picture of Cliff and you, that would be very special.

All my best, to a caregiver who cared so deeply from her heart,
Greg

Good morning, JoAnne—

I'm glad to hear you made it home safely. Snow moved in last evening and I'm sure the roads are icy. I got your voice mail and will call Precious Memories tomorrow. That is who needs to know. Thank you for the beautiful thoughts you sent about Cliff's passing. If we had to lose him, I am so glad it happened the way it did. I think we all hope for a peaceful transition like that, both for ourselves and for the ones we love. I hope I die with my head on the lap of my soul mate.

You are very articulate, and I look forward to your book. I want to thank you for being there for me too, this past year. I learned so much from Cliff, and I am grateful you always kept me up to date and kept in touch, even just to say hi. I think we made a good team! Please call if there is anything I can do for you. I will check in soon, just to say hi.

All my best,
Kim

Each time I read these e-mails, I cried new tears of missing Cliff. I was thankful that Kim and Greg would be there for me in the difficult days that lay ahead.

17
The Next Steps

I had a very difficult time in the days that followed. In an e-mail, Greg told me that it was normal to have roller-coaster feelings, many ups and downs; that it's been shown that losing a dog, and especially one like Cliff, could have the same emotional impact on someone as losing a child.

In a later conversation, he told me more about a VTH program called Family Support Services (FSS).

"I don't really like the name of the program," Greg said, "but I love the people. They help the doctors and staff through the hard times, and Kim and I have a session planned with them this week. I'm sure Cliff will be the topic. They are there for you, too," Greg continued, "and I can set up a session for you. They're like a Band-Aid for the hurting soul."

"Thank you for the offer, but I'm still not ready to talk to strangers," I said.

"Okay. Just keep it in mind," Greg said.

I decided to ask Greg about something that had been on my mind lately.

"Isn't it strange that from a medical standpoint, until December twenty-first, Cliff was still running, playing, and eating well?"

"Ah, that sounds like Cliff," Greg said. "He had tremendous joy in his life with you."

I smiled. *And he brought such joy to my life . . .*

When the autopsy results came back, Greg told me there were tumors throughout Cliff's body. Even in his precious heart. He said it was an absolute miracle that Cliff had done as well as he had before he got sick. That it was indeed a blessing he went to the angels in my arms.

The months following Cliff's death continued to be difficult. I went through times of second-guessing myself, second-guessing Cliff's care. *Had I done everything possible for him?* One day when I was at the VTH getting Jokonita examined, I ran into Ken, one of the oncology nurses who had often taken care of Cliff. It was the first time I'd seen him since Cliff's death. "How are you doing?" Ken asked.

"I'm okay," I replied. Something in my voice must have revealed my emotions. Ken gave me an intense look, and said, "You know, you did all you could for Cliff. There is nothing else you could have done." I felt my eyes start to fill with tears.

"Thank you," I said softly. "I know how much Cliff touched everyone. I am still seeing it now, months after his death. I feel very lucky that I was able to share Cliff's life with all of you." Ken smiled, and gave Jokonita a pat before he walked out of the exam room.

I continued to stay in contact with Kim and Greg, through visits to the VTH, phone calls, and e-mails. One day I told Greg that I was having a hard time trying to forget. "You will never forget—nor should you," Greg said. "Gradually, though, you *will* find a sense of peace with this circle of life. Cliff was a blessing to you. He survived beyond any reasonable expectation, beyond our wildest dreams."

I nodded, tears in my eyes.

"I know that you needed—and deserved—more time. But try to let this remind you that each day is a blessing that should be celebrated," Greg urged. "Each day we lose by weeping over things is a day lost, one which will never, ever be given to us again. This is what I have learned from my patients and friends who have passed away. I hope that Cliff's final and greatest lesson for you will be similar. While Cliff is not physically with us anymore, we will always have Cliff with us in spirit—each day, every day, *always*."

While Greg continued to support me, he also kept encouraging me to speak to Family Support Services. "There's no way Kim and I could do our jobs without the help of the folks at FSS," Greg said. "Veterinarians deal with death issues five times more often than physicians do. We deal with losses on a weekly basis, and we rely on the people at FSS for support.

"It upsets Kim and me that you continue to refuse this service. We want you to heal emotionally, as rapidly as possible. We don't want you to get stuck in an abnormal grief process. Grief is not very different from a physical hurt. If we break a bone and it is not set properly, it will not heal well. The same is true for grief; if it's not handled correctly, you will not be able to heal and move on with your life," Greg said.

I felt that he was pushing me away, pushing me toward FSS. I was so consumed with my grief that I was not thinking clearly. I had become more dependent upon Greg and Kim since Cliff's death, and I was clinging to what we had shared. I did not want to talk to someone at FSS. I wanted to talk to Greg and Kim. For some reason, I thought being with them would help keep Cliff's memory alive. I didn't realize then that only *I* could keep Cliff's memory alive. Being with Greg and Kim would not bring Cliff back to me, which was what I really wanted. I was not dealing with the reality of his death. I was getting stuck, just as they suspected.

In March, I got the news that Greg was going on sabbatical to France for a year. I did not take the news well. It was bad enough that Kim was finishing her residency. I knew she would be leaving soon, and I was prepared for that. I knew she would be taking a job somewhere else, but most likely would still be in the United States. I could not imagine Greg being so far away. What if I needed to talk to him? What if I needed to see him? He again encouraged me to seek the help of FSS. My only thoughts were: *How could strangers possibly understand what I was feeling?* Greg and Kim were the only ones who could really understand, because we'd lived through it together.

Right before Cliff died, Greg had told me that he had been the guy in the back all along. He'd known Cliff from the beginning. It hurt him to be the bearer of bad news in the last chapter of Cliff's life, and he wished he hadn't had to fill that role. It was uncomfortable for both of us. "You're part of our family, and you always will be. We're here to help and support you in any way possible," Greg said. And then, smiling, he added, "I'm afraid you're stuck with us—and we're happy to be stuck with you. But as your friends, we just want what's best for you."

His words finally got through to me, and I agreed to seek the help of FSS (which has since been renamed the Argus Institute for Families and Veterinary Medicine). I told Greg and Kim that it would be easier for me to communicate with the FSS staff via e-mail, as I was not yet ready to sit down and talk to anyone in person. Kim said she would ask Teri Nelsen at FSS to contact me. Teri did, saying she understood that I had been hesitant to utilize their services. She told me that this was not unusual, and she was there whenever I wanted to talk, in person or through e-mail.

We e-mailed for a few weeks, and then one day when I was at the VTH, I felt brave enough to stop by her office. I didn't know exactly how I would talk to her, but I thought it was time to try. By now I was not only dealing with Cliff's death, but also with the reproductive concerns I was experiencing with Jokonita, and the separation anxiety I was feeling with Kim and Greg both leaving. Teri assured me that it was very normal to develop a dependency on those who had provided care to Cliff. She told me that Kim and Greg were worried that I was getting trapped in the grief process.

During my first face-to-face session with Teri, I did not say much. I had a hard time talking about Cliff's death. She didn't try to push me. She let me go at whatever pace was comfortable for me. Sometimes I could hardly speak without tears. She assured me that Kim and Greg would still be there for me, but that they were not equipped to provide me the help I needed. I realized that I had put them in a difficult position: I had become too dependent upon them. I felt bad, because I'd never meant for that to happen.

I understood then that I *did* need the help of FSS. I had been stumbling through the grief process, and not doing very well on my own. I continued to see or e-mail Teri, and as the weeks turned into months, things slowly improved. I was still in a great deal of pain, but I was starting to feel better, becoming stronger each day. I accepted the fact that Kim and Greg were leaving. I came to realize that what Cliff and I had shared, through his life and through his death, had taught me a lot about myself. Living through this with him *had* made me a stronger person, and at the same time, a kinder and more compassionate one.

I was ready to move on.

18
Life as We Know It

I eventually found a new resting place for Cliff's ashes. My first purchase was a handmade brown pottery vase with a lid, discovered at an artisan's shop in Fort Collins. Unfortunately, once I got it home, I realized it was too small. I then decided on a simple, dark brown wooden box, with a lid and black metal hinges.

When it was time to transfer the remains, I carefully opened the floral box from the crematory, not knowing what to expect when I looked inside. I found his ashes tightly wrapped in a clear plastic bag, labeled with his name and weight. I carefully removed them, thinking how odd it was to see him in this form. Suddenly, I felt I understood why some people chose to sprinkle their loved one's remains back onto the earth.

First, I laid a small green towel in the bottom of the box and gently wrapped it around the bag of ashes—the green representing the soft grass he loved to rest on after playing outside. Then, inside the box I placed his brass choker collar, some beautiful blue feathers from a Steller's jay, a rose, and some photos of him. I wanted him someplace where I would see him often, so I placed the box on the center of my dresser, in the bedroom. On top of the box I set a few angel figurines.

This simple wooden box would be his final resting place, and I knew that it would accompany me often on my trips back and forth to Pennsylvania. I continued to add treasures to the box. Although I didn't know it then, months later, almost a year after Cliff's death, I would find myself writing a poem to commemorate his life and my love for him.

THE FEATHERS OF A HAWK

Eleven months and fifteen days
have helped to ease the pain;
reminders of your death,
a life not lost in vain.
A hawk no longer breathing,
its wings of feathers fold;
a simple wooden box,
now all the memories hold.

Mementos of our life,
the most precious gifts of all,
that day I stared death in the face,
now gifts from the sky do fall.
Your spirit still surrounds me,
through reminders of our life
things once so simple,
I no longer see as strife.

I weep at times,
and long to hold you close to me
In life comes death, and in death comes life,
if only we can see . . .
No other soul has touched my soul,
like that of yours gone by
through rays of sun, and moonlit skies,
I often wonder why.

Like feathers from this fallen hawk,
now added to your box
symbols of a regal life,
with instincts, keen as a fox.
Your death taught me life,
but what a price to pay—
one day we'll be together . . .
you'll be waiting for me that day.

More than a year after Cliff's death, Teri asked if I would come in and talk to a group of senior veterinary students about my experience with Cliff and his battle with cancer. While I knew it would be difficult to talk about what had happened, I agreed to do it. Since Cliff's death, I had found it much easier to write about it than to verbalize what I had gone through.

I did not prepare anything ahead of time, as Teri had indicated it would be a question-and-answer session with a small group of students. It was difficult at first, but when it was over and done with, I was glad I'd shared our story with them. Each time I wrote or talked about it, another piece of me healed. I felt I could finally say, in all honesty, that I was no longer stuck in my grief.

I thought of something Narda had recently told me—that after Cliff's initial diagnosis, the doctors had never expected him to live more than a few weeks. I was shocked when I heard this, thinking to myself, *But I'd always expected him to live.* In hindsight, I realized that I had never asked for a time frame; I had just assumed he would survive. I think this allowed me to keep an open mind and an open heart—and most of all, to never give up. After sharing this with Narda, she was quiet for a moment. Then she said, "This has been quite a spiritual journey for you." *How was it,* I wondered, *that she was able to see something inside me that I had only recently recognized myself?*

For during the past months, I had come to realize that Cliff had indeed taught me several important lessons: how to have the courage to move on; to not fear my fear; to embrace and accept things I have no control over; to love unconditionally. And, his most important lesson— to believe that miracles *can* happen. He had taught me well, and I hoped that wherever he was now, he could see the changes in me—changes that he had helped to create. He was much more my teacher than I was his.

Daily now when I am on the mountain, behind our Colorado home, I pass by Cliff's tree, the large aspen where Dick had so lovingly carved Cliff's name many years before. I pause by the tree, place my hand over the carving, and then place it over my heart. I glance up to the sky and whisper *I love you. I will always love you.* A place where before, I'd only felt sadness, I now felt gratitude, peace, and a deep and abiding love.

As the sun fades and darkness appears, I utter these few words: *Good-bye . . . I'll be back tomorrow.*

Afterword

More than four years have passed since the day Cliff went to heaven—December 31, 2001. After many unsuccessful inseminations, it was determined that Jokonita had cystic ovaries; they needed to be removed, and she was never going to be able to have Cliff's puppies. There is still enough of Cliff's sperm banked for eight more inseminations, and when the timing is right, I will get another female to breed.

A little over a year after Cliff's death, I got a new German shepherd puppy named Drake. He was flown over from Germany when he was twelve weeks old, and it was soon determined that he had a condition known as megaesophagus (mega-e).

The esophagus is the tube connecting the throat to the stomach. Normally when food is swallowed, it passes through the esophagus and enters into the stomach very quickly. When a dog has mega-e, the esophagus is enlarged, and the food tends to lie in the lower portion of the esophagus, not entering the stomach as quickly as it should. The largest risk in a mega-e dog is regurgitating some of the food and aspirating it into the lungs. This can cause aspiration pneumonia, a very serious, life-threatening illness.

After trying several different feeding regimens, I finally found one that works best for Drake: mixing his canned food with some water in a blender, to the consistency of a runny milkshake. I feed him this mixture from an elevated bowl, and mealtime is followed by some moderate exercise. This method allows the food to enter his stomach at a much quicker rate, with less chance of regurgitation.

His German family had named him Happy, because he was the happiest puppy in the litter. I had always wanted to name Cliff's firstborn male Drake, after the location of the VTH. So, Happy became Happy Drake, now known simply as Drake. He is now a beautiful three-year-old, weighing in at 75 pounds. He stands a whole head taller than Jokonita, and will always be on the lean side. Because of the mega-e, he does not receive any table scraps, which in the long run will aid in keeping him at a healthy weight. With careful feeding and management of the mega-e, Drake can live a long and healthy life. Every scare we have with an episode of regurgitation reminds me again of how precious each day is.

Jokonita, who is now nine and a half years old, raised Drake as her own; romping and rolling around on the floor together has helped to keep her young. It brings me great joy to see her sharing with Drake the same type of love she shared with Cliff. Although dogs love to be part of the human family, they also need companions of their own.

Living through cancer with Cliff gave me more patience, and equipped me well to raise a special-needs puppy. Together we are all a family. Cliff's pictures are still found throughout the house. My nephew Chase, who was two years old when Cliff died, is now six. When he looks at the pictures, he says, "That's Cliff. He's not here now—he's in heaven." I still sleep with Cliff's purple fleece blanket each night. I wonder if it was Cliff, my spirit in the sky, who sent Drake to me, to fill the void created by his death.

Thank you, Cliff. One day I will see you again. I miss you, and I love you.

COLORADO STATE UNIVERSITY
JAMES L. VOSS VETERINARY TEACHING HOSPITAL
www.csuanimalcancercenter.org

Over twenty-five years ago, Dr. Ed Gillette and Dr. Stephen J. Withrow established a cancer program at Colorado State University. Since that time, Dr. Withrow has led the Animal Cancer Center (the Robert H. and Mary G. Flint Animal Cancer Center) team to world prominence. The ACC's mission is to improve prevention and treatment of cancer in animals and humans, and the center has trained more veterinary oncologists than any other veterinary institution. It is the only veterinary cancer group to have more than twenty-five consecutive years of funding from the National Cancer Institute. Since the 1960s, Colorado State University's College of Veterinary Medicine and Biomedical Sciences has conducted innovative cancer research and provided state-of-the-art treatment for companion animals. Over the years, their work has also led to advances in the treatment of human cancers.

Dr. Withrow led a successful campaign to build a new facility for the center in 1998, raising $9.3 million for a new wing on the Veterinary Teaching Hospital. Dr. Withrow has gained international status and acclaim for his impressive career in animal cancer research, including groundbreaking efforts that have benefited both companion animals and humans. Among his many contributions to cancer research and treatment, Dr. Withrow developed a limb-sparing technique to treat osteosarcoma, a malignant bone tumor in dogs. This technique revolutionized treatment of this disease and has been widely adopted in human cancer centers.

The Animal Cancer Center (housed in the James L. Voss Veterinary Teaching Hospital) has pioneered numerous surgical, radiation therapy, and chemotherapy procedures for animals with cancer. Along with treatment and research, teaching is a key component of their mission. The center treats up to 2,000 pets a year with cancer and handles a volume of 10,000 appointments. The center is also home to the Argus Institute for Families and Veterinary Medicine, a unique center that studies the human-animal bond and provides grief resources to pet owners.

For more information about the CSU Animal Cancer Center, contact Paul Maffey, director of development for the Colorado State University College of Veterinary Medicine and Biomedical Sciences, at (970) 491–3932.

DR. GREGORY K. OGILVIE
CALIFORNIA VETERINARY SPECIALISTS (CVS)

Founded in 2000, California Veterinary Specialists (CVS) is one of the nation's leading providers of advanced multidisciplinary medical services for animals in need of critical emergency care and treatment of serious acute and chronic illnesses. Their specialty and critical care hospital network includes 24-hour, 365-day-a year state-of-the-art facilities serving San Diego County and the Inland Empire counties of Riverside and San Bernardino. Unlike other emergency and specialty veterinary groups that operate as separate businesses under one roof, they take an innovative team approach. Their experienced specialists in emergency, critical care, internal medicine, surgery, oncology, radiology, cardiology, and ophthalmology work together as one unit to provide the best integrated veterinary care available.

Angel Care Cancer Center for Animals
www.cvsangelcare.com

The CVS Angel Care Cancer Center for Animals is a center of hope, compassion, and healing, offering innovative treatment options for the whole patient, using a combination of medical, surgical, radiological, nutritional, physical, and supportive options. Their experienced team provides unmatched treatment and care while engaging in ongoing clinical research to explore new diagnostics and treatments in the fight against cancer. They work closely with primary care veterinarians, and their goal is to do everything possible to win the fight against cancer, while ensuring that the treatment is healing, not hurting.

Special Care Foundation for Companion Animals (SCFCA)
www.specialcarefoundation.org

Based in San Diego's North County, the Special Care Foundation for Companion Animals (SCFCA) was established in 2003 by Dr. Gregory K. Ogilvie, a world-renowned oncologist at California Veterinary Specialists (CVS). Before joining the team at CVS, Dr. Ogilvie was a tenured professor, internist, head of medical oncology, and director of the medical oncology research laboratory at Colorado State University. He has been awarded $5 million in research grants, and recently spent a year on sabbatical, teaching and developing new, innovative cancer therapies at the Université François Rabelais medical school in Tours, France.

The SCFCA is a nonprofit organization, and was created to provide philanthropic support for the development of promising treatments for cancer and other illnesses. Their mission is to celebrate the human-animal bond and enhance the quality of life of animals and people through compassionate care and a combination of medical, nutritional, and supportive options. The Foundation works hand in hand with a number of state-of-the-art facilities including CVS and their Angel Care Cancer Center, providing the opportunity to translate research findings into an active applied setting.

Funding for the Foundation is received from private and corporate sources whose donations, sometimes given in memory of an animal that has passed away, help to empower compassionate research and assist in the care of seriously ill animals on behalf of loved ones that could not otherwise afford such services. The Foundation also aims to provide financial assistance to care for animals in the wake of natural disasters such as earthquakes, floods, and fires.

For more information about the CVS Angel Care Cancer Center for Animals and Special Care Foundation for Companion Animals (SCFCA), contact Dr. Gregory K. Ogilvie at (760) 734-4433.

DR. KIMBERLY A. SELTING
UNIVERSITY OF MISSOURI-COLUMBIA
www.cvm.missouri.edu/oncology

Upon completing her oncology residency at Colorado State University, Dr. Selting achieved board certification in the specialty of oncology. She went on to join the faculty at the University of Missouri-Columbia, where she is currently an Assistant Professor of Oncology. The University of Missouri houses The Veterinary Medical Teaching Hospital (VMTH), a state-of-the art teaching and medical service facility. Faculty and students in the VMTH diagnose and treat more than 16,000 patients annually. Besides serving as a clinical laboratory, the VMTH provides specialty services to animal owners, including emergency and cardiovascular medicine and surgery, ophthalmology, neurology, orthopedic surgery, advanced imaging techniques, and oncology.

The VMTH has been involved in treating and studying animals with cancer as part of the medicine service since its inception. Dr. Dudley McCaw oversaw the treatment of animals with cancer for many years, and after the addition of Dr. Carolyn Henry in 1997, a separate oncology service was established. Since 2002, the service has grown with the addition of Dr. Kim Selting and more recently, Dr. Jeff Bryan. Currently three residents are being trained for board certification in oncology. The mission of the Oncology Service is to provide state-of-the-art, compassionate cancer care for animals, and in the process, to teach veterinary students, interns, and residents about safe and proper diagnostics and treatments.

With a caseload of twenty to twenty-five cases per week, dogs and cats with many kinds of cancer are treated, including lymphoma, osteosarcoma

146

(bone cancer), and carcinomas. In addition to providing standard-of-care treatment options for companion animals with cancer, the VMTH developed the Oncology Clinical Trials Service in 2003, to facilitate small animal patient participation in clinical trials to investigate new and promising cancer therapies. As part of a pioneering effort in radiopharmaceuticals, the UMC-VMTH oncology team is involved in trials evaluating Samarium-153-EDTMP, a bone-seeking radiopharmaceutical, for the treatment of bone cancer. Other research efforts include studies in epidemiology and proteomics of lymphoma and the genetic basis of breast and other cancers, evaluation of new drugs and chemotherapy protocols for treatment of lymphoma and leukemia, bladder, breast, skin, oral, and bone cancer, and techniques for earlier detection and improved imaging of many tumor types.

The Barkley House
www.barkleyhouse.missouri.edu

A fund-raising campaign is currently under way to build The Barkley House, the first Ronald McDonald House–type facility for families traveling to care for sick pets. The Barkley House will provide temporary lodging for animal patients and their families. Located near the Veterinary Medical Teaching Hospital, the compassionate, home-like environment will help to lessen anxiety for both pets and their families. Veterinary students will have additional opportunities to enhance their client-communication skills, and Barkley House will serve as a prototype for similar facilities at other veterinary referral centers.

For more information and to donate to The Barkley House or other oncology programs, contact: Greg Jones, Director of Development, College of Veterinary Medicine, University of Missouri-Columbia, W-203 Veterinary Medicine Building, Columbia, Missouri 65211, (573) 882–0548, or toll-free (888) 850–2357.

Resources

ACUPUNCTURE

Narda G. Robinson, DO, DVM, DABMA

American Academy of Veterinary Medical Acupuncture (AAVMA)

Department of Clinical Sciences

Colorado State University Veterinary Teaching Hospital

300 West Drake Road

Fort Collins, CO 80523

(970) 495–1918

www.aavma.com/contact.html

AMERICAN CANCER SOCIETY

www.cancer.org

**ARGUS INSTITUTE FOR FAMILIES
AND VETERINARY MEDICINE**

(formerly Family Support Services at the CSU VTH)

College of Veterinary Medicine & Biomedical Sciences

Colorado State University

(970) 297–4143

www.argusinstitute.colostate.edu

CANCER RESEARCH / DONATIONS—ONLINE GIVING

California Veterinary Specialists Special Care Foundation:

www.specialcarefoundation.org

Colorado State University

http://veterinarymedicine.colostate.edu/index.asp

University of Missouri

http://www.cvm.missouri.edu/oncology/waystogive.htm

CANINE REPRODUCTION / SPERM BANKING
Dr. Sheri L. Beattie
Brighton Animal Clinic
180 E. Bromley Lane
Brighton, CO 80601
(303) 659–2472
www.coloradoicsb.com

COLORADO STATE UNIVERSITY
VETERINARY TEACHING HOSPITAL (CSU VTH)
Dr. Stephen J. Withrow
Animal Cancer Center / James L. Voss Veterinary Teaching Hospital
Colorado State University
300 West Drake Road
Fort Collins, CO 80523–1620
Phone: (970) 221–4535
www.csuvets.colostate.edu/
www.csuanimalcancercenter.org

FAMILY SUPPORT SERVICES AT THE CSU VTH
See Argus Institute, above.

FLOWER ESSENCES
Flower Essence Society
www.flowersociety.org

HILL'S PET NUTRITION—PRESCRIPTION DIET CANINE N/D
www.hillspet.com

HOMEOPATHY

National Center for Homeopathy

801 North Fairfax Street, Suite 306

Alexandria, VA 22314

Phone: (703) 548–7790

Toll-Free: (877) 624–0613

E-mail: info@homeopathic.org

www.homeopathic.org

IP-6

American Cancer Society Article on IP6 (1998)

www.cancer.org/docroot/NWS/content/NWS_3_1x_IP6.asp

DR. GREGORY K. OGILVIE

California Veterinary Specialists

100 North Rancho Santa Fe Road, Suite 133

San Marcos, CA 92069

Phone: (760) 734–4433

E-mail: cvs@sbcglobal.net

www.cvsangelcare.com

www.specialcarefoundation.org

PET INSURANCE

www.petcareinsurance.com

www.petinsurance.com

www.petshealthplan.com

http://vetmedicine.about.com/cs/diseasesall/a/sickpetnomoney.htm

http://vetmedicine.about.com/cs/insuranceinfo/a/pethealthinsura.htm

PET LOSS
www.argusinstitute.colostate.edu
www.in-memory-of-pets.com
www.petloss.com
www.pet-loss.net
www.vetmedicine.about.com/od/lossandgrief/

REIKI AND ANIMAL COMMUNICATION
Dr. Brenda McClelland
Fort Collins, CO
www.energyworkdoctor.com
www.holistic-online.com/Reiki/hol_Reiki_home.htm

DR. KIMBERLY A. SELTING
University of Missouri, Columbia
Clydesdale Hall
379 E. Campus Drive
Columbia, MO 65211
www.cvm.missouri.edu

VETERINARY CANCER SOCIETY
www.vetcancersociety.org

WHEAT GRASS:
Ann Wigmore Natural Health Institute
www.annwigmore.org

About the Author

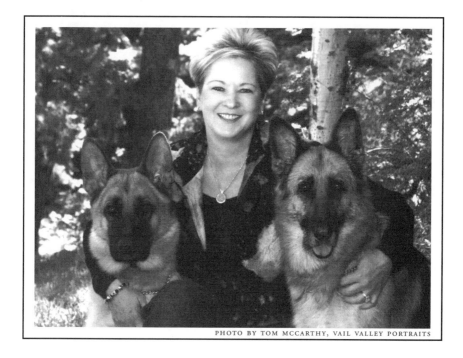

PHOTO BY TOM MCCARTHY, VAIL VALLEY PORTRAITS

Born and raised in a small town in Pennsylvania, JoAnne is the fourth of nine children. Her lifelong fondness of animals deepened when she met Cliff, who not only became a part of her family, but a part of her heart.

Because of her love of the outdoors, she now divides her time between two homes, one in Pennsylvania and the other in the Colorado Rocky Mountains. Her immediate family includes her husband Dick, stepson Blake, two cats, Tigger and Spooky, and the German shepherds she adores—Drake and Jokonita.

Her perfect day is spent in the company of those she loves, both two-legged and four-legged.